A New Ethic of 'Older'

Through its themes of subjectivity, surgery, and self-stylization this book critically examines the cultural constraints and incitements that shape the practice of cosmetic surgery by older people. The book problematizes anti-ageing discourses to provide a nuanced descriptive, ethical, and political reading of 'older' identity politics nested within the contemporary ethico-political terrain of self-care.

A New Ethic of 'Older' aims to de-territorialize the 'older' subject from normative discourses of ageing and theorize becoming 'older'. Evidence of an active cultural politics of 'older' emerges from the critically reflexive engagement of older people with cosmetic surgery. This engagement constitutes a 'cutting critique' of ageing discourses enmeshed in an aesthetic mode of subjectivation that underpins 'a new ethics of old age'.

The book will appeal to those in the fields of Cultural Gerontology, Ageing Studies, Critical Psychology, Sociology, and Cultural Geography. The methodological approach will be of interest to academics and students exploring the application of Foucault's work on care of the self to contemporary contexts and practices.

Bridget Garnham is a Research Fellow in the Centre for Social Change within the School of Psychology, Social Work, and Social Policy at the University of South Australia, Australia.

Routledge Key Themes in Health and Society

Available titles include:

Turning Troubles into Problems
Clientization in human services
Edited by Jaber F. Gubrium and Margaretha Järvinen

Compassionate Communities
Case studies from Britain and Europe
Edited by Klaus Wegleitner, Katharina Heimerl & Allan Kellehear

Exploring Evidence-based Practice
Debates and challenges in nursing
Edited by Martin Lipscomb

On the Politics of Ignorance in Nursing and Healthcare
Knowing ignorance
Amélie Perron and Trudy Rudge

Empowerment
A critique
Kenneth McLaughlin

The Story of Nursing in British Mental Hospitals
Echoes from the corridors
Niall McCrae and Peter Nolan

Living with Mental Disorder
Insights from qualitative research
Jacqueline Corcoran

A New Ethic of 'Older'
Subjectivity, Surgery and Self-stylization
Bridget Garnham

Forthcoming titles include:

Social Theory and Nursing
Edited by Martin Lipscomb

Identity, Ageing and Cultural Adaptation
Understanding longevity in crossdisciplinary perspective
Simon Biggs

A New Ethic of 'Older'

Subjectivity, surgery, and self-stylization

Bridget Garnham

Routledge
Taylor & Francis Group
LONDON AND NEW YORK

First published 2017
by Routledge

2 Park Square, Milton Park, Abingdon, Oxfordshire OX14 4RN
52 Vanderbilt Avenue, New York, NY 10017

Routledge is an imprint of the Taylor & Francis Group, an informa business

First issued in paperback 2019

British Library Cataloguing in Publication Data
A catalogue record for this book is available from the British Library

Library of Congress Cataloging in Publication Data
Names: Garnham, Bridget, author.
Title: A new ethic of "older" : Subjectivity, surgery and self-stylization / =Bridget Garnham.
Description: 1 Edition. | New York : Routledge, 2016. | Series: Routledge key themes in health and society | Includes bibliographical references and index.
Identifiers: LCCN 2016011112 | ISBN 9781472414601 (hardback) | ISBN 9781315565002 (ebook)
Subjects: LCSH: Aging--Psychological aspects. | Aging--Moral and ethical aspects. | Surgery, Plastic. | Self-perception.
Classification: LCC BF724.55.A35 G37 2016 | DDC 306.4/613--dc23
LC record available at https://lccn.loc.gov/2016011112

ISBN: 978-1-4724-1460-1 (hbk)
ISBN: 978-0-367-34908-0 (pbk)

Typeset in Times New Roman
by Taylor & Francis Books

Contents

	List of tables	vi
	Acknowledgement	vii
1	Introducing a new ethic of 'older'	1
2	*Designing* 'older' rather than denying ageing	30
3	The fractured 'older' subject at the limits of 'ageing'	57
4	To look *better*, not younger	73
5	Ageing *dis*gracefully and *becoming* 'older'	99
6	Concluding cuts	126
	Index	135

Tables

2.1	Chronology of media texts (1992–2008)	47
2.2	Participant profiles: 'older' people who have undergone cosmetic surgery	49
2.3	Participant profiles: cosmetic surgery practitioners	51

Acknowledgement

I am very grateful to all the people who agreed to be interviewed for this book and for the support that cosmetic surgeons provided which made the research possible. I recall the 'older' people whose perspectives inspired this work with both gratitude and admiration for their vibrancy, forthrightness, and goodwill. I hope this tale does you justice.

My deepest gratitude goes to Vicki Crowley for supporting me through troubled times, for challenging and inspiring me in unfamiliar realms of thought, for liberating my writing voice, and for encouraging my learning and progress. I am humbled by your ethical sensibilities.

During the writing of this book I have enjoyed the mentoring and scholarly engagement of Lia Bryant. Your support has enhanced my self-belief and your example has inspired my courage. I am so grateful for the fun and friendship we share through our mutual passions for critical and transformative scholarship, writing and, of course, shopping.

The arguments offered up in this book were honed and hotly debated through good-humoured intellectual sparring with my friend and interlocutor, Jodie George. I am most grateful for your critical engagement and support in developing this work. I believe I may now rest my case.

I am grateful to Colleen Deery for the artwork that beautifully resonates with the themes of this book and permission to reproduce this piece on the front cover.

The manuscript for this book took shape within the scholarly space afforded to me within the Centre for Social Change and benefitted from a culture of writing practice and the emotional support, solidarity, and friendship of my colleagues.

The time to write this book was a gift from my mum, Mary Garnham granted through care for my children. I am deeply grateful for your support and recognition that writing this book was important to me. You have always inspired, encouraged, and supported my learning and scholastic achievement. For this, I dedicate this work to you.

//

1 Introducing a new ethic of 'older'

Beginning to rethink 'older'

Radical transformations to cultural representations of 'older'[1] and rapidly diversifying embodied experiences of 'older' ages constitute a torrent of social change in advanced capitalist democracies across the globe. Structurally, these nations are ageing due to falling fertility rates and the large cohort of baby boomers who are reaching older ages with greater life expectancies; in terms of both mortality and how to live a life in old age. Increasing in numbers and heterogeneity, in these hyper visual media-mediated societies, older people are becoming progressively visible in advertising, television and film (see Krainitzki, 2014; Marshall and Rahman, 2015). In entertainment news, older people feature in stories that challenge traditional images and meanings of older age and older bodies. For instance, as I write this introduction, a story that surfaced across national news and social media platforms over the past week has been that of Eileen Kramer, who at 100 years of age is to feature dancing in a music video for Sydney-based musician Lacey Cole. A dominant narrative across these mainstream media platforms is that older people are becoming actively engaged – with their careers, their social and intimate relationships, leisure pursuits, fitness, travel, and no end of possibilities for spending their accumulated wealth and time. This broadening array of possibilities in the social and cultural milieu of our present suggests new ways of 'doing older' that provide both the impetus and focus for this book.

The substantive focus of the book emerges from the observation that increasing numbers of older people are choosing to undergo cosmetic surgery.[2] In much academic thought on cosmetic surgery, the notion that surgery is used to produce a younger or more youthful appearance in an ageist society means that cosmetic surgery is judged as an ageist practice counterproductive to challenging societal ageism (e.g., see Bayer, 2005; Hurd Clarke and Griffin, 2007; Hurd Clarke, Repta and Griffin, 2007; Gilleard and Higgs, 2000). Similarly, in media reporting, cosmetic surgery is often associated with moral judgement for 'denying ageing' and refusing to be 'old' or 'elderly' (e.g. Crawford, 1999; Ryan, 2001). Through their repeated elicitation in this ethical problematization, discourses of 'ageing' have become normalized and operate to constitute an essentialist conception of age and 'older'. Taking inspiration from ideas about the materiality of the body as 'cultural text' (see Grosz, 1994; Foucault, 1976) and body modification as discursive re-inscription (see Chen and Moglen, 2006; Featherstone, 1999; Pitts, 2003), this book problematizes this normative and essentialist rendering to ask the question anew, what is being written in the flesh of the 'older' body and what does this mean for 'doing older'?

Through its themes of *subjectivity, surgery and self-stylization* the cultural constraints and incitements that shape the practice of cosmetic surgery by older people are explored in this book. Discourses of 'ageing' and 'anti-ageing' as they permeate cosmetic surgery practice among older people are problematized to offer what Sedgwick (1997) might consider a 'reparative reading'; one that evokes conditions of artistry and freedom of self-stylization that exceed the normative limitations of 'ageing'. Such a 'reading' offers:

> a theoretical analysis that has a political meaning – I mean an analysis that has meaning for what we want to accept, refuse and change of ourselves, in our actuality. In short, it is a matter of starting out in search of a different critical philosophy: a philosophy that does not determine the conditions and limits of a knowledge of the object, but the conditions and undefined possibilities of the subject's transformation.
>
> (Gros, 2005: 526)

By engaging with questions of how interpretations and thought concerning 'older' and cosmetic surgery might be transformed, the analytic practices of this book therefore engage 'politics as an ethics' (Foucault, 1984b: 375). This approach entails 'the interaction between theory and practice' whereby 'thinking and acting are connected in an ethical sense, but one which has results that have to be called political' (Rabinow, 1984: 376–377). Following Braidotti (2002: 3) such an approach can usefully be conceptualized as a 'cartographic reading of the present in terms of cultural, political, epistemological and ethical concerns'. In the chapters to follow, encounters between theory and textual data drawn from research interviews and media reports are used to problematize discourses of ageing and offer a reading contextualized by 'ethopolitics' in which *becoming* 'older' is subject to self-stylization through cosmetic surgery. In other words, this book offers the interpretation that older people who engage with cosmetic surgery are *designing* 'older' rather than denying ageing.

Doing 'older' differently

The ways in which people aged in their mid-sixties and beyond are 'doing older' connects with 'older' subjectivities. As feminist scholars pursuing post-essentialist conceptions of the subject have shown, subjectivity can be thought of and analysed in terms of the processes that produce self-hood (e.g. Bartky,

1988; Butler, 1990; Fraser, 1997; Grosz, 1994). These processes are social, draw on cultural discourses for meaning and are historically contextualized. Subjectivity is therefore multiple, contingent and fluid. What this tells us is that changes to the ways in which older people understand and express identity are not only personal but shaped by social, cultural and historical contexts and conditions that give rise to norms and expectations about what it means to be an 'older' person and how to live a life in old age. Older people navigate these norms and expectations in forming a social identity by taking up, resisting and contesting particular discourses that constitute 'older' subjectivities in ways that are desirable and undesirable. This way of thinking about identity formation resonates with conceptions of identity as a 'project' (Giddens, 1991) and the 'point of *suture*' between multiple subjectivities (Hall, 1996: 5). As only one dimension of identity, 'older' intersects with other social categories of identity and difference. Feminist proponents of intersectionality approaches have examined gender, race, class, sexuality 'etc.' (see, for instance, Hulko, 2009; Valentine, 2007; Villa, 2011; Yuval-Davis, 2006) but a sustained engagement with ageing is yet to occur (cf. Calasanti and King, 2015). However, the intersectional possibilities among various axes of social identity, embedded in shifting social, cultural and political contexts, provides fertile ground for heterogeneous and dynamic productions and performances of 'older' subjectivities.

Doing 'older' is not only a social and cultural phenomenon but an embodied identity. The significance of the material body in social and cultural processes of social identity formation emerged in scholarship that provided a theoretical and analytic nexus between corporeality and discourse (e.g. Featherstone, 1991; Grosz, 1994; Lester, 1997; Shilling, 2003; Turner, 1991). This work produced conceptions of identity as inscribed upon and read from the material surface of the physical body. In these accounts, embodiment is central to understanding subjective experience of identity. In terms of 'older', the physical and chronological ageing of the body, rendered intelligible through corporeal signifiers and a cultural matrix of norms relating to age and appearance, have been essential to the social constitution and recognition of the 'older' subject. The inscription of 'age' in the flesh of the body has thus been pivotal to the ways in which 'older' is experienced and performed. Early critical scholarship from beyond the margins of traditional gerontology sought to reveal how essentialist biomedical discourses constitute ageing as physical decline and decrepitude and inscribe these meanings in old and aged bodies in ways that devalue, stigmatize and marginalize 'older' people (e.g. Gullette, 2004; Hepworth, 2003; Katz, 1996; Tulle-Winton, 2000). This work has also sought to locate the 'problems' of ageing in the social body by problematizing the ageism that renders aged and older bodies undesirable (e.g. Biggs, 2002; Hurd Clarke, 2001).

Whilst the materiality of the body can be understood as socially inscribed, the body also provides a site for exercising agency and expression of the self. Rather than 'inert' or 'docile', as Grosz (1994: xi) suggests, bodies 'function interactively and productively. They act and react. They generate what is new, surprising and unpredictable'. Through its generative capacity and unpredictability, the body is therefore 'able to be used in potentially infinite ways, according to infinite variable cultural dictates' (Grosz, 1994: 146). So whilst biomedical discourses have over-inscribed the 'older' body, the materiality of old and aged bodies provides a site for exploring the emergence of marginalized, previously subsumed or newly emerging cultural discourses. In particular, practices of 'body modification' (e.g. Featherstone, 1999; Pitts, 1999; Pitts, 2003; Sullivan, 2001) such as cosmetic surgery provide an opportunity to explore bodily inscription according to the discourses that inform those practices and the social, cultural and political contexts in which those practices are embedded and take shape.

In the context of body modification practices, cosmetic surgery has a privileged history of critical analysis within feminist scholarship. Much of this literature problematizes cosmetic surgery according to oppressive patriarchal structures enacted through a male 'gaze' and the production of heteronormative femininity (e.g. Blum, 2003; Gagne and McGaughey, 2002; Gilman, 1999; Morgan, 2009; Wolf, 1990). This work, as Pitts-Taylor (2009b: 120, 119) suggests, constitutes cosmetic surgery as an oppressive normalizing practice and the women who undergo cosmetic surgery as 'self-hating and self mutilating' victims of 'politically oppressed consciousness'. The condemnation of cosmetic surgery and women who chose to have cosmetic surgery fed into the structure–agency debates that polarized feminist literature. Concerned by the positioning of women as 'cultural dopes', scholars such as Davis (1995, 2009) and Gimlin (2000, 2006) responded by asserting women's 'agency'. They argue that rather than trying to vainly achieve standards of beauty, the women in their empirical studies were motivated by psychical suffering and the desire to achieve a 'normal' appearance. Bordo (1998, 2009) countered Davis's claims with the argument that notions of 'freedom' and 'choice' have their surface of emergence in consumer culture and are thus overdetermined by a larger patriarchal structure that ensures cosmetic surgery becomes a reasonable choice. The problem and impasse that both sides of the structure–agency debate produce, as Pitts-Taylor (2009b: 121) argues, is that 'they insist on the centrality of women's subjectivity in problematizing cosmetic surgery'. What Pitts-Taylor suggests, is that these accounts centre an essentialist subject by probing 'deep motives, mental health or political consciousness' to explain the 'truth' of cosmetic surgery.

Contemporary post-essentialist feminist scholars such as Fraser (2009), Heyes (2007), Jones (2008) and Pitts-Taylor (2007, 2009) argue that cosmetic surgery discourse is neither external to the subject, to be internalized or refused by a pre-existing self, nor a practice for unmediated self-expression. Rather, the practice of cosmetic surgery is implicated in the very processes of *becoming* a subject and possible forms of subjectivity in Western societies and cultures. In terms of agency, to borrow from Fraser (2009: 104), the 'subject does not "exercise" an agency implanted by culture which she or he then possesses, rather the subject is produced through the various forms of agency available at any given moment'. This point resonates with Foucault's, and later Butler's, conception of power and subjectivation whereby the operation of power '*enacts* the subject into being' (Butler, 1997: 13). Foucault's accounts of power radically problematize conceptions of agency and resistance. Following Foucault, Butler (1997: 15 emphasis in original) argues that the subject is 'the *condition of possibility* for a radically conditioned form of agency'. The subject is therefore enacted through agency, but that agency does not provide unfettered freedom. Rather, the possibilities for 'freedom' are shaped by social, cultural and political contexts and practices that precede the subject. In addition, however, as Butler (1997: 12) further explains, the power that produces the subject is not necessarily the same as the power wielded by the subject as an effect of agency. Through enacting its own *becoming*, 'the subject eclipses the conditions of its own emergence; it eclipses power with power' (Butler, 1997: 14). Butler (1997: 15) concludes that 'agency exceeds the power by which it is enabled'. Through this notion of 'exceeds', Butler suggests that whilst relations of power form the conditions of existence these never 'contain' the subject, leaving open the question of *becoming*. Following Foucault's and Butler's theorization of subjectivation and conceptualization of agency thus enables a nuanced analysis of power as it is implicated in the processes and practices by which the subject is formed. Relating this back to cosmetic surgery, as Pitts-Taylor (2009: 122) suggests, 'we must think of the meanings of bodily practices like cosmetic surgery as neither solely internal nor external but rather as intersubjective'. What she is suggesting is that the subject is shaped through the practice of cosmetic surgery by acceptance, resistance and transgression of a multiplicity of dynamic social, cultural and political discourses. In this book, the theoretical insights offered by this scholarship compels examination of the possible forms of subjectivity available to 'older' people and how the practice of cosmetic surgery is engaged to navigate, adapt or adopt subject positions located within social, cultural and political conditions of possibility.

Cosmetic surgery is largely enmeshed, constituted and enacted within the discursive framework of consumer culture (Elliott, 2008). This means that the meanings of cosmetic surgery largely emerge from an 'aesthetics of existence' within which the 'continual shaping, fashioning and presentation of the body' is paramount (Besley and Peters, 2007: 41). In this system of thought, the body is a commodity and 'project' (Shilling, 2003) that imitates other 'lifestyle projects' associated with DIY and 'renovation'. Jones (2008: 1) refers to this broader lifestyle phenomenon as 'makeover culture' and argues that 'cosmetic surgery is makeover culture's quintessential expression'. For consumer culture theorists like Bauman (2008) and Baudrillard (1998), commodities exist within a semiotic system and consumption operates to transfer the meanings attached to the commodity to the consumer. Moreover, the force inciting the consumer to purchase commodities for what they signify is largely desire rather than lack or need. The freedom within this system to desire and choose what is desirable enables consumers to reflexively stylize identity. As Featherstone

(2007: 81) elaborates, 'one's body, clothes, speech, leisure pastimes, eating and drinking preferences, home, car, choice of holidays, etc. are to be regarded as indicators of individuality of taste and sense of style of the owner/consumer'. However, the freedom to choose as an individual consumer right is simultaneously an ethical responsibility. Refusing to engage with consumption, or the refusal to choose, is constituted as a choice and as a choice it signifies something about the consumer – such as a lack of taste, style or status. In the context of the aestheticization of everyday life, consumer culture and practices of consumption therefore provide 'sites of distinction' (Gilleard and Higgs, 2000: 8) for a multiplicity of cultural positions in relation to 'older'. Amid this growing cultural abundance many 'older' people reflexively engage in acts of consumption and fashion lifestyles to provide form and self-expression to social identity. The engagement of older people with cosmetic surgery thus provides an interesting case study for exploring the self-stylization of contemporary 'older' identities. In addition to providing insight into the phenomenon of older people who engage with cosmetic surgery, this focus also pursues new possibilities for problematizing the ontology of 'older'.

Critique of 'older'

As a sociological category of identity and difference, the ontology of 'older' has not been subjected to the same radical critique and theoretical transformation that scholars have enacted with categories of gender, sexuality and race. As Cruikshank (2008: 149) points out:

> it seems curious that the identity "old" has not undergone similar transformation in age studies. The social construction of aging is widely acknowledged, but the expansive and revisionist thought on "woman" and "gay" finds few parallels with "old" as an identity.

Whilst scholarship within ageing studies has explored and illuminated the ways in which 'ageing' is discursively constructed and shaped by social, cultural and political conditions (e.g. Featherstone and Wernick, 2005; Gilleard and Higgs, 2000; Gilleard and Higgs, 2013; Gullette, 2004; Hepworth, 2003; Katz, 2005; Powell, 2006; Powell, 2011), this has had limited impact in terms of transforming theoretical and cultural conceptions of 'older'. Equally, feminism has been charged with ageism and failing to critically engage with questions of ageing and older women. One reason for this lacuna, as Gilleard and Higgs (2013: 4) suggest, pertains to the 'absence of a viable social movement promoting the interests of older people'. Social movements generally gain momentum through collective moral outrage and become galvanized by political aims that seek to remedy issues of injustice, oppression and social marginalization. It is evident that older people have been subjected to oppressive effects of power through the medical pathologization of ageing, social policies that limit autonomy and cultural stigma (e.g. Gilleard and

Higgs, 2000; Gullette, 2004; Hepworth, 2003; Katz, 1996; Powell, 2006). Oppressive characterizations of 'older' people as potentially senile, physically decrepit, sick, unattractive, needy, vulnerable, socially reclusive and lonely have deeply shaped possibilities for the subjective experience of 'older' (e.g. Bennett and Gaines, 2010; Sánchez Palacios, Trianes Torres and Blanca Mena, 2009; Smith et al., 2011). Yet this has not translated into a cohesive or highly visible social collective geared towards social activism.[3] Cruikshank (2013: 6) suggests that the powerlessness of older people may manifest as a docile colonized personality, 'pinned down by the category "old"'. Moreover, Gilleard and Higgs (2000: 3) assert that 'Old age itself is not a site that is seriously contested or challenged. It remains a period of life that is excluded, marginalized or institutionalized'. The approach taken in this book contends that whilst there may not be a highly visible and cohesive social movement, there is evidence of an active cultural politics of 'older', that 'older' is indeed being contested and challenged and that cosmetic surgery, as a practice of self-stylization, provides a site for exploring this activism.

Similar to the identity politics of other social groups that seek to 'reclaim ways of understanding their distinctiveness that challenge dominant oppressive characterizations' (Heyes, 2009: n.p.), the cultural politics of 'older' entails struggles around how 'older' identities are understood. In all identity politics, the point of contest centres on the ways in which subjectivities are 'put into discourse' (Foucault, 1976: 11) and the ensuing effects of power that shape subjective experience and either provide opportunities for freedom or delimit autonomy. At present, discourses of 'ageing' dominate the 'grid of cultural intelligibility' (Butler, 1990) that render 'older' subjectivities intelligible. The problem here is that current discourses of ageing are reductive and operate to limit the subjective experience of 'older' in oppressive and stigmatizing ways. Thus, the central contention of this book is that discourses of ageing are the heart of the problem for the identity politics of 'older'.

The trouble with 'ageing' for becoming older

Ageing is both problematized and taken-for-granted in thinking about older people. Indeed the two concepts are so tightly intertwined that 'ageing' often stands in for 'older' with no disruption to comprehension. This is evident in academic scholarship in 'ageing' studies, where the substantive focus is on older people, as well as social policy where the focus of government offices, such as the Department of Ageing and Aged Care and Office for the Ageing in Australia, are the social, health and welfare needs of older people. Yet ageing and older are not the same. We are ageing all our lives and so it is somewhat perplexing that ageing assumes such prominence during later stages in the lifecourse. As Baars (2009: 87) writes:

> It may be one of the main gerontological paradoxes that all human beings age, but at a certain moment in their lives they are labeled as

> "aged" or "older" (older than whom?) and their living beyond that point as "aging". The expressions "aged" and "aging" are without any further explanation used as references to an abnormal group, although these expressions actually indicate a universal and continuous process of living in time.

So what is it about ageing once we are assigned the status of 'older' that is any different? What after all *is* ageing? As soon as this foundational question is posed in such a way that suggests ageing may not have an unyielding ontological security, a plethora of additional questions pour fourth. Is ageing a central pillar of social identity like gender, sexuality, and race? But, how is ageing theoretically and phenomenologically different to social constructs like gender or race since transition from one life stage to another is a normative expectation of ageing? Whilst discourses and cultures of ageing have been problematized for some time in the academic literature (e.g. Cruikshank, 2013; Gilleard and Higgs, 2000; Gullette, 2004; Katz, 2005; Katz and Marshall, 2003; Powell, 2006), a sustained critique and theorization of the ontology of ageing and the possibilities and limitations of this for thinking about 'older' is only beginning to emerge (e.g. Riach, Rumens and Tyler, 2014; Tulle, 2008b). Knowledge of ageing however, has a long history that is interwoven with and emerges in particular systems of thought including gerontology as the traditional site of knowledge of 'ageing', the multidisciplinary field of 'ageing studies' and most recently, cultural gerontology. Through the discourses produced by these disciplines, these systems of thought extend into social, political and cultural sites of practice related to ageing and older people.

Biomedicalization of ageing

Given their status as scientific, 'biomedical accounts occupy a privileged and dominant position' in terms of producing the truth about 'ageing' (Twigg, 2004; Wahidin and Powell, 2003). However, in terms of basic knowledge of the biology of ageing, biogerontology, unlike many of its colleagues in the natural sciences, is yet to determine the fundamental mechanisms of its object of study. Indeed, Gems (2011: 108) claims this to be 'one of the greatest remaining challenges to science'. Despite not having definitively addressed the question, in biological terms, of what ageing *is*, biomedical discourses dominate understandings of ageing in the health and social sciences, much of ageing studies and of course gerontology and geriatrics. These understandings emerge from an essentialist framework of ageing as a universal, intrinsic property of physical organic bodies which change over time. In biomedical discourse these changes, conceptualized as 'ageing', are both normalized and pathologized. The ageing of 'young' bodies is normalized through understandings of physical maturation and development whereas the ageing of 'older' bodies is constituted in terms of mental and physical decline and decrepitude that is both normal, in that it is to be expected, and pathological because it deviates from youthful norms. Through its framing as pathological decline, biomedical discourse extends further to constitute ageing as a 'disease' for which a cure or treatment should be sought (Gems, 2011; Grey, 2007). As Gems (2011: 109) states 'from the perspective of modern biogerontology, there is little to distinguish biological ageing from a disease state'. The conflation of ageing and disease means that chronic illness and physical dysfunction become normalized as part of ageing for 'older' people but bear no discursive connection to ageing for younger people. Indeed, the 'early onset' of particular illnesses is considered 'premature' and thus tragic when these illnesses manifest in younger bodies. Whilst epidemiological research may demonstrate that the prevalence of physical dysfunction and disease increases with age, this is not the same as saying that these are synonymous with or central characteristics of ageing or the experiences of 'older' people. Equally, this discursive framework problematizes youthful bodies with physical dysfunction and disease as non-normative or abnormal.

Socio-political regulation of ageing

By providing a legitimate evidence-base of true and valid knowledge of ageing and older people, the biomedicalization of ageing extends into other discursive frameworks (Gilleard and Higgs, 2000; Katz, 1996; Powell, 2006). One site in which the outworking of this discourse has powerfully shaped possibilities for older people is within social policy and practice. Gilleard and Higgs (2000: 126) elaborate on this connection in their assertion that 'The "physiological neediness" of the ageing body has been seen as justifying many of the policies concerning retirement, social security, health and welfare that have evolved over the first half of the last century'. Given that definitions of 'older people' in Western democracies have traditionally been based upon social policy and practice, particularly retirement and social pension scheme eligibility, this has led to a conflation of 'ageing' and 'older' such that the biomedicalization of ageing has colonized what it means to be 'older'. Through this colonization, 'older' is 'made evident in its bodily manifestations' (Tulle-Winton, 2000: 78) of decline and decrepitude.

Given the apparent 'physiological neediness' of the ageing body, 'older people' are 'socially regulated within demographic and policy categories of risk and dependency' (Katz and Marshall, 2003: 3; Tulle-Winton, 2000; Warren, 1998). Elaborating on the government of 'risk', Rose (2001: 7) writes:

> there are actuarial or epidemiological strategies that seek to reduce aggregate levels of risk across a population. There are strategies for the management of high risk groups. And, increasingly, there are strategies based on identification of, and preventative intervention for, risky individuals.

Observing how medical and political discourse intersect in the politics of risk, Powell (2006: 138) states that 'medical and political discourse contribute to a subterranean coherence, which may help to explain their co-existence. Each offers a view of aging while downloading "risk" and uploading "responsibility" onto aging subjects'. Or, in Rose's (2001) words, 'biological identity generates biological responsibility'. In terms of the physical decline and decrepitude that constitutes biological ageing, 'older' people are subjected as 'risky individuals' which legitimates preventative medical surveillance and intervention and, increasingly, ethical requirements for self-care.

Most recently the social 'risk' posed by older people has been framed through the economic threat to social sustainability accompanying population ageing. Posed as a global 'challenge' (Phillipson, 2013) the problematization of demographic ageing occurs through the prism of neoliberal political economy in advanced Western democracies. Sociologists and social theorists in ageing studies have focused on how this socio-political framework has provided a surface of emergence for the 'active ageing trilogy: healthy, productive and successful ageing' (e.g. Asquith, 2009; Mendes, 2013: 175; Moulaert and Biggs, 2013; van Dyk, 2014). This trilogy represents a proliferation of social discourse on ageing well where 'well' stands in for good health, social productivity and economic security. The political-economic imperative for these discourses is considered to be driven by the need to reduce social welfare expenditure and contribute to national economic growth.

As Gilleard and Higgs (2000: 38) observe, the inauguration of these active ageing discourses have enacted the social and cultural transformation of 'older' 'from pensioners to senior citizens to third-ager'. The newly retired or flexi-retired 'third-ager' is (re)presented as wealthy, physically healthy and active and enjoying high levels of wellbeing and life satisfaction (see, for example, Featherstone, 1995; Gilleard and Higgs, 2000; Katz and Laliberte-Rudman, 2005; Katz and Marshall, 2003). Through the deployment of 'successful', 'positive', 'productive' and 'active' ageing discourses, neoliberal governmental strategies position third-agers as individually responsible for shaping positive experiences of 'older'. Publically circulating images of the 'wellderly' suggest later life to be a time of active leisure, wealth and lifestyle consumption. Positioned according to these contemporary sociopolitical discourses, the 'new generation of retired people finds itself in a position of greater potential agency' (Gilleard and Higgs, 2002: 370). However, this agency is shaped by new normative expectations about how to age and be 'older' in contemporary neoliberal societies. Juxtaposed, new and traditional discourses of 'ageing' generate tensions and contradictions in the ways in which 'older' is constituted and experienced in contemporary neoliberal consumer society (see, for example, Gilleard and Higgs, 2000; Katz and Laliberte-Rudman, 2005; Katz and Marshall, 2003; Paulson and Willig, 2008; Powell, 2006). The nature of these tensions is captured by Katz and Marshall (2003: 12) who state, 'on one hand [older people] are led to understand that the expectations for them to be active (including sexually active), mobile, autonomous, experimental, knowable, networked, and consumer-niched will contribute to their care, well-being, visibility and inclusion within public worlds of participation and care'.

However, 'on the other hand, retired and older people are governed within lifestyle profiles allied with neoliberal and antiwelfarist agendas to restructure dependency and problematize their ageing bodies and identities as vulnerable, risky, and in need of self-vigilance'.

By exploring the outworking of these tensions and contradictions, scholars have critiqued the limitations of contemporary 'positive' discourses of ageing to argue that 'successful ageing' simply 'masks' rather than supersedes the biomedicalization of ageing (Powell, 2006). As Higgs et al. (2009: 689) suggest, these new discourses of ageing mean that 'ageing and the hazards of growing older form another arena in which the autonomous self is expected to act and make the right choices'. The means by which individual health consumers are expected to take responsibility for their ageing, is through the consumption and practice of 'healthy lifestyles' to 'avoid the undesirable ravages of ageing' (Hodgetts, Chamberlain and Bassett, 2003: 426). The outworking of this discourse for older people renders ill health, disability, chronic disease, and any change to physical capacity, the result of individual 'ageing' and thus failure to age 'successfully'. Through the discourse of 'healthy lifestyles', 'ageing' is constituted as an accumulation and consequence of individual 'choices' made across the lifespan. This operates to preclude social determinates of health that are enmeshed with housing, employment, education and income (Mendes, 2013) and 'failure' to age well becomes gendered, classed and raced in alignment with stratified access to social and economic capital (e.g. Castillo et al., 2010; Koutsogeorgou et al., 2014; Ziegler, 2012).[4]

Critical ageing studies and cultural gerontology

Through the dominance of the biomedicalization of ageing, the scientific traditions within the field of 'ageing studies' typically reduced ageing to an organic property of the body and this led to a restricted, self-perpetuating focus of scholarship. Gilleard and Higgs (2000: 194) contest this restricted focus stating:

> Our argument is not that there are no poor old people, nor that retired people do not, in some cases, experience significant limitations in managing their daily lives...Rather we are arguing that through emphasizing the plight of the poor and disabled within the retired population, an academic and popular discourse has been perpetuated that makes these phenomena the very essence of ageing and ageing studies.

By pursuing a limited vision of ageing, the diversity and multiplicity of ways in which 'older' people experience and make sense of their lives was traditionally neglected in ageing studies. However, following the 'cultural turn', critical scholarship emerged that used philosophical interventions shaped by the 'posts' to explore how 'ageing' is culturally constituted and the effects of this on the social identity of 'older' people (e.g. Cruikshank, 2003; Featherstone and Wernick, 2005; Gullette, 2004; Gilleard and Higgs, 2000; Gilleard and Higgs, 2013; Hepworth, 2003; Katz, 2005). As Gilleard and Higgs (2000: 13) argue, the substantive contribution of this work has been towards 'seeing ageing as a cultural process, moving from the view that ageing is something that happens to people toward recognizing it as something individuals have to engage with'. This extends from the broader projects of social theory that theorize social identity as a reflexive project of the self (Giddens, 1991), discursively constituted (Foucault, 1982), embodied (Grosz, 1994) and performative (Butler, 2004). This critical scholarship has fractured the boundaries of ageing studies and created pathways into a plethora of research possibilities for understanding heterogeneous experiences of ageing, the ageing body and ageing subjectivities as contextualized within social, political and cultural conditions. The rapid maturation and development of this field over the last decade has recently consolidated and established itself as the discipline of 'cultural gerontology' (Twigg and Martin, 2015). Emerging themes in this field of scholarship include consideration of what an ageing body 'can do' (Fox, 2005) including sport, body building and human movement research (Dionigi, 2006; Phoenix and Smith, 2011; Tulle, 2008a; Tulle, 2008b), research exploring sexuality and sexual expression of older people (e.g. Fileborn et al., 2015; Montemurro and Siefken, 2014; Rowntree, 2014; Wada, Hurd Clarke and Rozanova, 2015), the generational ageing of 'youth' sub-cultures (Hodkinson, 2011; Hodkinson, 2013), and research that focuses on aesthetics and preferences through the prism of ageing and in connection to older people (e.g. Twigg and Majima, 2014; Ward, Campbell and Keady, 2014). This scholarship is also engaging in radically new ways with more traditional themes from gerontology including dementia (Buse and Twigg, 2015; Twigg, 2010; Kontos, 2015), care (Fine, 2015) and falls (Katz, 2015).

In terms of developments in understanding the ontology of ageing, a body of recent literature has emerged that examines discourses or the embodiment of ageing in relation to intersecting axes of social identity and fracture including gender, sexuality and class (e.g. Calasanti and King, 2015; Domínguez-Rué, 2012; Hilário, 2015; Hurd Clarke, Bennett and Liu, 2014; Lodge and Umberson, 2013). Indeed, Gilleard and Higgs connect the centrality of the embodiment of age and ageing to the advent of a 'new ageing'. Whilst informed and shaped by broader theoretical developments in sociology and cultural studies concerning ways of thinking about the body, agency and the formation of identity, critical scholarship engaged with 'new ageing' will need to grapple with its own challenges given the peculiar nature of ageing. As Gilleard and Higgs (2013: 4) suggest:

> As an inherently dynamic process, ageing threatens to destabilize whatever settlement might be negotiated between the particular embodied identities represented by gender, race and disability and the institutional practices and cultural narratives of operating in society.

Whilst gendered, sexed and raced identities might be continually constituted and dissolved, the inculcation of norms means that individuals generally experience a stable sense of self. As Butler (1990: xv) has described in relation to gender, 'what we take to be an internal essence of gender is manufactured through a sustained set of acts, posited through the gendered stylization of the body'. The 'sustained set of acts' refers to the process of performativity which occurs according to 'a repetition and a ritual' that gives appearance to a naturalized and stable gender identity. Given that ageing is 'inherently' dynamic, it therefore sustains an 'unsettling influence' on embodied identity (Gilleard and Higgs, 2013). 'Ageing' thus presents a somewhat elusive ontology, but one that must be considered in terms of its reference to age.

Age

As Cruikshank (2013: 209) observes, 'our chronological age is both meaningful and meaningless'. This is because chronological age is laden with social and cultural meanings but has no essential nature. Tulle (2008b: 7) develops this idea further through Bourdieu's theorizing and her suggestion that 'we could conceive of age itself acting as a structure guiding our social location and our dispositions – in other words acting as habitus'. This is a significant contribution to theorizing age and ageing in a way that locates possibilities for lived experience beyond the ageing body. As Tulle (2008b: 7) suggests, this approach entails 'paying attention to the set of dispositions which are open to us as we age, particularly as they involve particular choices, decisions, strategies and aspirations which coincide with one's position in the social structure'. 'Age' therefore provides possibilities for particular norms, expectations or dispositions to become internalized by the subject while foreclosing others or rendering them distasteful, undesirable or subject to social sanction. Think for instance about how age norms operate to govern socially acceptable modes of conduct in relation to sexual relations, birth and parenting of children, formal education, fashion and appearance, access to finance and economic systems and so on. Of course, as soon as age-related norms are rendered visible, their conditional nature, as shaped by social, cultural and historical contexts, also emerges in concert with possibilities for resistance and transgression. Age related norms, the contexts in which they operate and the available possibilities for agency can thus be understood as comprising a 'habitus' that provides 'ageing' with meaning and structure that appears self-evident and natural.

As Thomas et al. (2014: 1570) suggest, 'age has become a reified system of classification and a pervasive organizing principle with significant effects'. The most significant effect is that through ordinary forms of social organization and structure, 'age' has become naturalized and normalized as a central 'truth' of the subject. This 'truth' is embedded in everyday life as we are socially and culturally compelled to make careful and accurate statements that record and reinvoke the date on which we were born and the passage of years. To lie about one's age is typically regarded as futile, as age constitutes an interior essence that poses as 'real'. Culturally we are captivated by the game of guessing a person's 'real' age based on physical appearance and confounded when someone appears 'younger' or 'older' than their appearance would suggest. Essentialist discourses of ageing therefore install age bound norms that are restrictive and reduce the potential for being 'otherwise'. Seeking a parallel to heteronormativity, Freeman (2010) has developed the concept of 'chrononormativity' to problematize social expectations anchored by stages in the lifecourse that produce normative or viable subjectivities. Through its engagement at the level of discourse however, such an approach does not extend into the fleshy body to problematize the corpo-*reality* of age.

The body: age, ageing, and appearance

Much of the ageing studies literature that has focused on the body in terms of age and ageing has traditionally done so within the parameters of critiquing the biomedicalization of ageing and structural ageism (e.g. Biggs, 2002; Featherstone and Wernick, 2005; Hepworth, 2003; Tulle-Winton, 2000; Wahidin and Powell, 2003). This literature weaves in and out of analytic focus in relation to discourses that constitute the ageing body, lived experiences of ageing embodiment and appearance of the ageing and aged body. However, a dominant discourse that emerges from across this literature is one that 'constructs aging bodies as "problem bodies"' (Öberg, 2003: 103). In terms of appearance, the ageing body is discursively imprisoned by the dichotomy of 'youthful' and 'aged'. This mode of thinking about the presentation and appearance of the body is so heavily inscribed by discourses of the ageing body that it becomes virtually impossible to think outside these parameters. Academic discourse on 'youthful ideals' provides a centrifugal point which anchors understandings of bodily appearance. This, of course, has proven useful for demonstrating how the undesirability of the aged and ageing body is inaugurated and sustained. However, it has also foreclosed upon possibilities for alternative and more nuanced analyses of bodily appearance and age. The discourse on 'youthful ideals' is in itself a normative universal discourse that fails to account for diversity or age trajectories in appearance that run in contradiction to its field of visibility. For instance, there are 'youthful' bodies that are not 'ideal' and there are bodies that are rendered more desirable and closer to the 'ideal' as they age.

The discourse of 'youthful ideals' also oversaturates ways of thinking about certain practices of body modification through a naturalized reinscription of 'ageing'. This means that some practices for altering the appearance of the body, including some cosmetic surgery techniques, are constituted and problematized in terms of 'anti-ageing', denial of ageing, masking the signs of age, creating an appearance of 'agelessness' or a more 'youthful' look (e.g. Ellison, 2014; Hodgetts, Chamberlain and Bassett, 2003; Hurd Clarke, 1999; Hurd Clarke and Korotchenko, 2010; Katz and Gish, 2015; Katz and

Marshall, 2003; Longino and Powell, 2004; Slevin, 2010). As Gilleard and Higgs (2000: 60) suggest, these practices are considered constitutive of an identity of 'staying young, choosing not to grow old'. In media and some academic discourses, 'older' people who engage in cosmetic surgery are almost singularly considered to be 'denying ageing'. Higgs et al. (2009: 699) argue for example, that 'anti-ageing medicine' including cosmetic surgery comprises practices of self-care that 'seek to overcome the ageing process or mask the signs of ageing'. These practices of body modification are thus subject to scholarly critique because they are considered to produce an appearance of 'non-agedness that further reinforces the undesirability and fear of old age' (Gilleard and Higgs, 2000: 81). The discourse of 'anti-ageing' in connection to practices of bodily appearance is so thoroughly entrenched in systems of thought in academic scholarship, consumer culture and mass media production that it is rarely problematized (cf. Twigg, 2012; Phoenix and Smith, 2011). This has meant that the focus of academic advocacy has been on social and cultural change oriented to valuing aged bodies and physical signifiers of 'ageing'. However, these efforts reinstate essentialist conceptions of the body in which the truth of age and 'ageing' is unproblematically signified in the fleshly surfaces and folds of the body.

Denying ageing or ageing norms?

The problem with claims about 'denying ageing' is that they are premised upon essentialist conceptions of 'ageing' and 'problematically construct a natural, essential, authentic body' (Pitts-Taylor, 2009: 121). In terms of the 'older' body, to borrow from Twigg (2004: 60), '[e]ssentializing discourses in relation to the body need to be replaced by ones that recognize its nature as a social text, something that is both formed and given meaning within culture'. Conceptualizations of the body as a surface or plane of signification can generally be traced to Foucault who describes the body as 'the inscribed surface of events…totally imprinted by history' (Foucault, 1984a: 83). What he suggests is that the materiality and comportment of the body are shaped and given meaning through practices of discursive inscription. Through these practices, power is invested in the 'text' of the body and operates to shape the way in which it is 'read'. Given this theorization of the body, the 'path to ageing "naturally" is highly problematic' since 'If there is no natural body, then there is no natural way to age' (Twigg, 2004: 63). If there is no natural way to age, then how can it be possible to deny ageing?

Drawing on Judith Butler's theoretical insights concerning gender, certain parallels can be made in terms of the effects a normative, essentialist rendering of 'older' has for individual experience. A central problem that Butler addresses in her work, is the operation of norms in the relationship between the subject and truth that delimit possibilities for being 'otherwise'. As Connolly comments in an interview with Butler (Butler and Connolly, 2000), 'the demand to secure a "true identity" or "a core" identity is entangled with ugly processes that close off the development of a plurality of identities on the same social field'. Butler illustrates and elaborates on this notion in her statement that:

> if a core gender contains the critical truth of gender, then it is possible to announce about another person that the truth of their gender is manifested by their acts or their appearances. This can be used to say that the truth of a masculine-looking woman is her core femininity – which she denies – or that the truth or a feminine-looking woman is her core femininity – which she affirms.

What Butler is suggesting here does not entail a refusal of the materiality or comportment of the body. Rather, what Butler insists, is that gender is a prescribed entity, inscribed upon and through the materiality and comportment of the body. Through its inscription, gender stylizes the body according to a 'critical truth' or core essence, in ways that exclude alternative ways of being and action. By drawing parallels with Butler's thought, it becomes possible to suggest that through its normative, essentialist rendering, the critical truth of 'older' is manifested through the acts and appearances of 'older people'. This can be used to say that a 'youthful' looking or acting 'older person' is denying their ageing – or less forcefully, is 'good for their age' – or that an aged appearance or manner of acting affirms the truth of ageing as physical decline. An essentialist core of 'older' thus enables norms to 'extend their own power to order the entire field of moral and political judgement' (Butler, 2001: 11). Through this structure and ordering, alternative possibilities for being and action are foreclosed and thus 'ageing' inaugurates limits to the ontology of 'older'. A critique and problematization of ageing norms is therefore imperative to the cultural politics of 'older'.

***Becoming* 'older'**

Through 'ageing' we become older. However, 'older' can also be understood as a socially and culturally defined stage in the framework of the lifecourse. This means that 'older' is relative and can only be understood in its relation to other stages – including infancy, childhood, youth and middle age. As a prescribed stage in the lifecourse, 'older' is bounded by chronological age but its onset is nebulous and dependent on which markers are selected to signify transition into this stage. Whilst the onset of 'older' is uncertain and shifting, its conclusion is finite and this apparent proximity with the inevitability of human mortality casts an ontological shadow over the possibilities for its cultural construction. (For theorizing of the 'fourth age' see: Gilleard and Higgs, 2010; Higgs and Gilleard, 2014; Sánchez Palacios, Trianes Torres and Blanca Mena, 2009.) 'Older' however, is not the only linguistic convention that refers to the final stage in the course of life. For the politics of identity, complex questions arise concerning the language and analytic categories used for representation. The array of choices materialize according to particular discursive frameworks and provide a political terrain to be navigated according to the benefits and dangers accorded to each. The elderly, the old, the aged, pensioners, retirees, third-ager, older people, young old, and old old are all terms that carry baggage consisting of values, symbolic meanings and connotations that exceed semantics, since they evoke particular relations of power and knowledge. In ageing studies, Gilleard and Higgs (2000) for instance, have rejected the designation of 'old age' in favour of 'cultures of ageing' arguing that this approach allows for multiplicity and flexibility as well as opportunity for viewing agency in terms of how individuals engage with the changes that occur with age. Here they assert that 'old age' cannot be easily reframed or transgressed since cultures of ageing are principally shaped by their resistance to old age. They retain this emphasis on ageing in their more recent text (Gilleard and Higgs, 2013) in which they consider intersections between ageing and embodied identity. In this text however, they acknowledge that 'new ageing' 'is as much a sociology of "not becoming" old as it is one of "becoming old differently"' (Gilleard and Higgs, 2013: 20). Cruikshank directly takes on 'old' as the object of analysis in her text but considers the ways in which social constructions of age and ageing intersect with gender, race and class to shape subjective experience within this stage of life. In an earlier piece, she contends that the category 'old' reflects a problematic essentialism given that its designation confers little special insight into the nature of those it signifies. This point raises the question as to whether 'old age' confers the same analytic cogency as gender, sexuality, class or race. But to attempt to answer that question is perhaps to miss the point. Again, Cruikshank (2008: 150) provides an interesting point for consideration:

> What if "old" is a fictive category, a convenient illusion far more relevant to the not-old than to those whose chronological age is thought to mean a great deal? What if the country of the old has no borders?

If the designation of 'old age' is not a fixed identity and does not confer particular meanings then its construction is opened up to a plethora of possibilities. Doing 'older' differently thus becomes a viable political alternative involving choice with respect to how to *become* older.

The idea of *becoming* 'older' allows engagement with the notion of transformation. This is a particularly suitable conceptualization since it is an identity category that inherently involves movement from one designation to another as those who were once youth become middle aged and then become older. Using 'older' to evoke notions of *becoming* also aligns this work with scholarship that attends to subjectivity as progressive and fluid (Braidotti, 2002; Grosz, 1999), formed and dissolved through multiple engagements with machinic assemblages (Guattari, 1995) or the effect of performative practices (Butler, 1990; Butler, 1997) . Such an approach is politically and ethically inspired in order to evade and reject essentialist discourses of 'ageing'. The significance of this is captured by Gilleard and Higgs's (2013: 31) argument that 'even as bodily ageing is re-imagined by the new ageing and in the narratives and performances of its still desiring subjects, agedness itself remains cast within old discourses and dividing practices of an earlier set of assumptions'. So the following chapters of this book are driven by a new question, one of how the subject *becomes* 'older'. To pursue this question entails exploring processes of identity work and lifestyling in later life as these are undertaken 'in' and 'through' the body and evoke forms, styles and values pertaining to 'older'. Such an approach provides scope and possibilities for understanding the formation of 'older' subjectivities that might illuminate research findings that show older age as a period of greater life satisfaction and wellbeing (e.g. Quéniart and Charpentier, 2012). In this cultural space, 'older' age might be rendered as 'inherently worthy, not requiring qualifiers like "positive" or "successful" to render it desirable' (Cruikshank, 2008: 151).

Introducing a new ethic of 'older'

To understand the constitution of 'older' subjectivities differently and explore examples of how 'older' is being transgressed and transformed according to new possibilities, this book considers old age a site for moral reflection. As with much contemporary theorizing in ageing studies, this approach decouples the object of study from earlier essentialist renderings guided by insights that social categories of age, gender, class and race are produced through a matrix of social, cultural and political discourses within a historical context. This means that old age, as a socially inscribed position in the life course, is given form through meanings that can undergo modification and transformation through time and vary according to their location in particular geographical and cultural contexts (see Gilleard and Higgs, 2013 for discussion of historical transformations). However, the premise of this book is that old age also needs to be understood as a site for subjective critical reflection and self-conduct within an ethical framework.

The enduring philosophical question of how to age well provokes and sustains the ethical problematization of old age. Reflecting on old age as a 'problem', diverse fields of thought situated in academic and scientific knowledge, social policy and organizational frameworks in concert with cultural representations, generate prevailing truths and norms about what it means to age well, be an older person and live a life in old age. From this problematization, moral ideals and cultural practices emerge that collectively form an ethic that gives form to a 'desirable old age'. At present, in neoliberal democracies, principles of 'ageing well', 'ageing productively', 'positive ageing' and 'active ageing', derived from social policy and academic discourses have recast older ages as a time of active leisure, wealth and lifestyle consumption for the ethically virtuous (see, for example, Featherstone, 1995; Gilleard and Higgs, 2000; Katz and Laliberte-Rudman, 2005; Katz and Marshall, 2003; Powell, 2006). The ethic constituted by these principles provides the values and ways of acting that individuals can meditate upon and engage with in order to shape the self as an ethical subject of 'old age'. Understanding the ethical formation of the 'older' subject is therefore critical to recognizing how old age can be a site for reflexive self-expression.

Much of the critical scholarship within aging studies has been oriented towards revealing how older people are subjected by relations of power connected to neoliberal political governance and consumer cultures (e.g. Asquith, 2009; Gilleard and Higgs, 2000; Katz and Laliberte-Rudman, 2005; Katz and Marshall, 2003; Laliberte Rudman, 2006; Powell and Biggs, 2000). As previously discussed, this literature offers critique of 'positive', 'successful', 'active' and 'productive' ageing that demonstrates how neoliberal governmental strategies position 'older' people as individually responsible for their health, financial and social security and overall wellbeing. As Katz and Laliberte-Rudman (2005: 140–144) observe, the 'new ageing' 'is built on the ethics and responsibilities of self-care'. However, in much contemporary scholarly discourse, 'older' is positioned at the centre of an ethical problematization in which self-care practices are considered constitutive of an identity of 'staying young, choosing not to grow old' (Gilleard and Higgs, 2000: 60). In this way, the discursive framework of 'ageing' envelops a myriad of practices including exercise, active leisure pursuits, clothing selection, use of make-up, hair dye and cosmeceuticals that for older people are rendered within the pursuit of 'youth' or maintaining 'youthfulness'. The outworking of this discursive positioning thus transforms the ethical reading of 'self-care' into one of 'anti-ageing'.

The interpretation of cosmetic surgery as a practice of 'self-care' and 'self-stylization' in this book draws insights from Michel Foucault's (1990a, 1990b, 1994, 2005) analyses of ethics in relation to sexuality in ancient Greek and Roman texts. Foucault was concerned with the normalizing power of modern Western modes of ethics, which through scientific knowledge anchored subjectivity in 'truth' so that sexuality became an essential nature of the self. He pursued analysis of the ancient Greek and Roman texts because they revealed an alternative aesthetic mode of ethical self-constitution anchored in a stylistics of existence rather than truth. This aesthetic ethic was dominated by the principle of 'care of self' which meant continually 'working on' or 'being concerned with' the self by engaging in practices oriented towards achieving an existence characterized by virtue and beauty (Foucault, 1994). Foucault, in his discussion of Seneca's writing, briefly mentions the significance of this ethic of the self for understanding 'older'. He writes:

> now that the care of the self must be practiced throughout life, but especially in adult life, now that the care of the self assumes its full dimensions and effects when one is fully adult, we see that the moment of the successful outcome and of the highest form of the care of the self, the moment of its reward, is precisely in old age.
>
> (Foucault, 2005: 108)

What Foucault is suggesting, is that the benefits of having taken care of oneself throughout life are realized in old age. Through the continual practice of taking care of the self, Foucault (2005: 110) suggests that it is possible to attain 'an ideal old age; an old age we produce, as it were, which we practice'. Given this conceptualization of an ideal old age, Foucault (2005: 109) suggests:

> Old age should not be seen merely as a limit on life, any more than it is to be seen as a phase of diminished life. Old age should be considered, rather, as a goal, and as a positive goal of existence. We should strive towards old age and not resign ourselves to having it come upon us one day. Old age, with its own forms and values should orient the whole course of life.

Whilst Foucault was writing about ancient Greek and Roman ethics, these ideas offer great potential for how we might begin to reimagine 'older' in contemporary contexts. Since Foucault died in 1984 prior to the advent of the increasing problematization of ageing and ageing populations we will never know how he might have brought these ideas to bear on reconceptualizing the ontology of 'older'. The chapters of this book therefore pursue a 'new ethics of old age' (Foucault, 2005: 110) by bringing Foucault's thought on ancient ethico-aesthetics into dialogue with contemporary social and cultural theory and empirical data. In doing so, the analysis in this book reveals a transgressive cultural politics that opens into new possibilities for shaping an 'older' identity and lifestyle with the potential to destabilize and transform understandings of old age by exceeding the discursive boundaries of 'ageing'.

Chapter 2, '*Designing* "older" rather than denying ageing', problematizes the normative rendering of the ontology of 'older' and the practice of cosmetic surgery by 'older' people through discourses of ageing. The chapter develops a theoretical approach to understanding cosmetic surgery that draws on Foucault's work and in particular his writing on ancient Greco-Roman ethics and care of the self. The chapter elaborates on the contention that whilst the principle 'know yourself' has dominated Western Cartesian ethics, 'care of self' offers potential for analysing somatic ethics in the context of the aestheticization of everyday lifestyles. Within these lifestyles, self-care enacted through practices of care for the body constitutes the ethical subject. To develop tools for analysing how the ethical subject is constituted within this regimen, the chapter attends to Foucault's conceptualization of the four folds of subjectivation: the ethical substance, mode of subjection, practices of self, and *telos.* Finally, the chapter engages with Foucault's suggestion that practices of 'care of self' are linked to critique of what we 'are' and provide a means for transforming the self. Cosmetic surgery can therefore be interpreted as a practice of the self that offers a site for examining the problematization and ethical self-stylization of 'older' identities.

Chapter 3, 'The fractured "older" subject at the limits of "ageing"', explores how a Cartesian ethics fractures the 'older' subject. Within this ethics the 'ageing' of the body generates a problematization of the relation between a subjective sense of the self and the corporeal body. Media texts and interviewees articulate this problematization in terms of dissonance between an 'aged' appearance of the body and an internal sense of an 'ageless' self. In academic literature, this problematization is conceptualized as the 'mask of ageing' and an outworking of the essentialism in Cartesian ethics. The chapter suggests that this mode of ethics constitutes the critical field (Probyn, 1993) in which the 'older' body and self are rendered intelligible in relation to the practice of cosmetic surgery. In this ethical domain, the self is constituted as 'authentic' through a mode of subjectivation associated with the hermeneutics of the subject and the 'older' body is problematized as the ethical substance and site for ethical work. This mode of subjectivation limits the ethic of the self in relation to freedom and aesthetic stylization. The analysis in this chapter reveals that the 'older' body is problematized as declining, deviant and surgically risky through normative discourses of ageing and that these discourses render features of the 'older' body abject to enable practices of surgical repair. From here, the central contention is established that the problem is not the 'older' body but the way in which it is rendered intelligible in relation to 'ageing'.

Chapter 4, 'To look *better*, not younger', problematizes the rationality of anti-ageing discourse inscribed in cosmetic surgery practice. It argues that anti-ageing discourse operates to differentiate certain practices of cosmetic surgery as 'anti-ageing' and differentially position 'older' consumers in relation to 'younger' consumers. This is a problem for the cultural politics of 'older' because anti-ageing discourses constitute cosmetic surgery as an ageist practice and 'older' consumers as denying ageing. Such a reductive reading of the body, in which age operates to norm appearance, retains a latent essentialism premised upon the constitution of the naturally ageing body. Privileging the discourse articulated by participants that cosmetic surgery is practiced to look *better* not younger, and following Pitts-Taylor (2009: 126), links the practice of cosmetic surgery to aesthetic concerns that matter because they are 'deeply superficial'. To elaborate the significance of, the discussion explores alternative rationalities inscribed in cosmetic surgery in relation to somatic ethics and a regimen of self-care. Reimagined as a practice of self, cosmetic surgery is discursively positioned at the nexus between technology for aesthetic enhancement (self-improvement), therapeutic intervention (self-fulfilment) and consumer choice (self-indulgence). Reading beyond technology, cosmetic surgery is embedded in the context of neoliberal consumer culture whereby ethical care of self occurs through self-fashioning an appearance and 'lifestyle' in the aestheticization of everyday life. The aesthetic and creative sensibilities that inscribe the practice of cosmetic surgery therefore provide possibilities for challenging and exceeding normative limitations concerning the appearance of the 'older' body.

Chapter 5, 'Ageing *dis*gracefully and *becoming* "older"', explores how the subjective experience of 'older' is reflexively fashioned to constitute the ethical self and problematizes the ethical and aesthetic principles of 'ageing gracefully' and 'mutton dressed as lamb'. The aesthetic style and grace associated with 'ageing gracefully' entails taking care of the self through practices that cultivate the body. However, the normative rendering of this principle suggests a passive acceptance of ageing 'naturally'. A cultural politics premised on 'ageing gracefully' is therefore limited by the essentialism of the natural body and will fail to transform the discursive framework that renders 'older' bodies undesirable. To overcome this problem, the chapter suggests problematizing 'youth' in aesthetics and developing a (re)inscription of 'older' bodies through desire and desirability. Drawing on participants' discourse to pose a counter politics of 'ageing *dis*gracefully' draws attention to the ways in which discourses can be seized in acts of voluntary insubordination to modes of subjection that constitute 'older'. This chapter further develops the central contention of the book that 'older' people want to look better not younger by exploring the ethical self-stylization of 'older' selves and lifestyles. It argues that this is more than an aesthetic preference and is embedded in interpersonal relations between self and Other and struggles around subjectivity to challenge, resist and subvert forms of subjectivity connected to being 'aged'. The chapter demonstrates that through creative self-fashioning of aesthetic sensibilities, 'older' is being opened up to new possibilities and practices in the context of contemporary ethopolitics that exceed the boundaries of ageist discourses.

Summary

A reflective surface of emergence for the cultural politics of 'older' is offered through an ethico-political interpretation that problematizes 'older' in relation to cosmetic surgery. Through a critique of the colonization of 'older' by 'ageing', this book argues that 'older' people engage with cosmetic surgery as an ethical practice of self-care, to *design* 'older' rather than deny ageing. In doing so it problematizes the essentialism that inscribes the ontology of 'older' in currently prevailing systems of thought. Practicing politics as ethics, the book intervenes in these systems of thought by opening up possibilities that exceed the limitations of 'ageing'. It establishes that when 'ageing' prefigures 'older' then 'older' always comes into view and is framed as a problem; a problem of decline, pathology and risk but also a problem of physical and social limitations and constraints. If 'older' has no essential nature then the limitations and constraints are imposed by a politics of truth that forecloses on possible identities and sensibilities. This book appeals for a reconceptualization of 'older' that opens cultural spaces for opportunity and possibility, desire and desirability; a reconceptualization that ethically engages the subjective experiences of 'older' people to illuminate the richness of the cultural texts and practices that 'older' people engage to stylize a mode of existence. Such a reconceptualization acknowledges that agency and freedom are preconditions for disciplinary power and neoliberal governmentality but also resistance, transgression and transformation.

Notes

1 Like Bytheway (2003) I use the term 'older' in an open sense to designate a stage in the lifecourse that follows 'middle-age'. It is also the term used in social policy in Australia where the research for this book was undertaken. For discussion of nomenclature refer to Mendes, F. R. 2013. Active ageing: A right or a duty? *Health Sociology Review*, 22, 174–185.

2 Media reporting, based on evidence from professional bodies like the British Association of Aesthetic Plastic Surgeons, suggests that this is a burgeoning demographic in their patient profile (e.g. The Canadian Press. 2002. More People 65 And Older Getting Cosmetic Surgery. 24th July.)

3 There have been social movements challenging the social exclusion of older people and age-based discrimination – for instance the Gray Panthers in the USA – but these have been limited in their momentum and capacity to drive social and cultural change.

4 The social determinates of health are being addressed within the current revisions of the active ageing framework WHO (2015).

References

Asquith, N. 2009. Positive Ageing, Neoliberalism and Australian Sociology. *Journal of Sociology*, 45, 255–269.

Baars, J. 2009. Problematic Foundations: Theorizing Time, Age and Aging. In: Bengtson, V. L., Gans, D., Putney, N. M. & Silverstein, M. (eds) *Handbook of Theories of Aging*. New York: Springer Publishing Company.

Bartky, S. 1988. Foucault, Femininity, and the Modernization of Patriarchal Power. In: Diamond, I. & Quinby, L. (eds) *Feminism & Foucault: Reflections on Resistance*. Massachusetts: Northeastern University Press.

Baudrillard, J. 1998. *The Consumer Society: Myths & Structures*. London: Sage Publications.

Bauman, Z. 2008. *The Art of Life*, Cambridge: Polity Press.

Bayer, K. 2005. Cosmetic Surgery and Cosmetics: Redefining the Appearance of Age. *Generations*, 29, 13–18.

Bennett, T. & Gaines, J. 2010. Believing What You Hear: The Impact of Aging Stereotypes upon the Old. *Educational Gerontology*, 36, 435–445.

Besley, T. A. C. & Peters, M. A. 2007. *Subjectivity and Truth: Foucault, Education and the Culture of the Self*. New York: Peter Lang Publishing.

Biggs, H. 2002. The Ageing Body. In: Evans, M. & Lee, E. (eds) *Real Bodies: A Sociological Introduction*. Basingstoke: Palgrave.

Blum, V. L. 2003. *Flesh Wounds: The Culture of Cosmetic Surgery*. California: University of California Press.

Bordo, S. 1998. Braveheart, Babe, and the Contemporary Body. In: Parens, E. (ed.) *Enhancing Human Traits: Ethical and Social Implications*. Washington DC: Georgetown University Press.

Bordo, S. 2009. Twenty Years in the Twilight Zone. In: Heyes, C. & Jones, M. (eds) *Cosmetic Surgery: A Feminist Primer*. Surrey: Ashgate Publishing.

Braidotti, R. 2002. *Metamorphoses: Towards a Materialist Theory of Becoming*. UK & USA: Polity Press.

Buse, C. & Twigg, J. 2015. Materialising Memories: Exploring the Stories of People with Dementia through Dress. *Ageing and Society*, 1–21.

Butler, J. 1990. *Gender Trouble: Feminism and the Subversion of Identity.* New York: Routledge.

Butler, J. 1997. *The Psychic Life of Power: Theories in Subjection.* Stanford: Stanford University Press.

Butler, J. 2001. *What is Critique? An Essay on Foucault's Virtue* [Online]. Available: http://eipcp.net/transversal/0806/butler/en [Accessed 25 May 2016].

Butler, J. 2004. Bodily Inscriptions, Performative Subversions. In: Salih, S. & Butler, J. (eds) *The Judith Butler Reader.* USA: Blackwell Publishing.

Butler, J. & Connolly, W. 2000. Politics, Power and Ethics: A Discussion Between Judith Butler and William Connolly. *Theory & Event*, 4, 28.

Bytheway, B. (2003). Visual Representations of Late Life. In: Faircloth, C. A. (ed.), *Aging Bodies: Images and Everyday Experience.* Walnut Creek: AltMira Press.

Calasanti, T. & King, N. 2015. Intersectionality and Age. In: Twigg, J. & Martin, W. (eds) *Routledge Handbook of Cultural Gerontology.* Oxon: Routledge.

Castillo, J. M. D., Navarro, J. E. J., Sanz, J. L. G., Rodriguez, M. M., Izquierdo, A. C. & Pines, D. D. H. 2010. Being Physically Active in Old Age: Relationships with Being Active Earlier in Life, Social Status and Agents of Socialisation. *Ageing and Society*, 30, 1097–1113.

Chen, N. N. & Moglen, H. (eds) 2006. *Bodies in the Making: Transgressions and Transformations.* Santa Cruz: New Pacific Press.

Crawford, P. 1999. Should be the Year of Facelift. *Sunday Tasmanian*, 30 May.

Cruikshank, M. 2003. *Learning to be Old: Gender, Culture and Aging*. Boston: Rowman & Littlefield.

Cruikshank, M. 2008. Aging and Identity Politics. *Journal of Aging Studies*, 22, 147–151.

Cruikshank, M. 2013. *Learning to be Old: Gender, Culture and Aging*. Plymouth, UK: Rowman & Littlefield.

Davis, K. 1995. *Reshaping the Female Body: The Dilemma of Cosmetic Surgery*, New York: Routledge.

Davis, K. 2009. Revisiting Feminist Debates on Cosmetic Surgery: Some Reflections on Suffering, Agency, and Embodied Difference. In: Heyes, C. & Jones, M. (eds) *Cosmetic Surgery: A Feminist Primer.* Surrey: Ashgate Publishing.

Dionigi, R. 2006. Competitive Sport as Leisure in Later Life: Negotiations, Discourse, and Aging. *Leisure Sciences*, 28, 181–196.

Domínguez-Rué, E. 2012. Mothers, Daughters and Midlife (Self)-discoveries: Gender and Aging in the Amanda Cross' Kate Fansler Series. *Journal of Aging Studies*, 26, 428–437.

Elliott, A. 2008. *Making the Cut: How Cosmetic Surgery is Transforming Our Lives*, London: Reaktion Books.

Ellison, K. L. 2014. Age transcended: A semiotic and rhetorical analysis of the discourse of agelessness in North American anti-aging skin care advertisements. *Journal of Aging Studies*, 29, 20–31.

Featherstone, M. 1991. The Body in Consumer Culture. In: Featherstone, M., Hepworth, M. & Turner, B. S. (eds) *The Body: Social Process and Cultural Theory.* London: Sage Publications.

Featherstone, M. 1995. Post-Bodies, Aging and Virtual Reality. In: Featherstone, M. & Wernick, A. (eds) *Images of Aging: Cultural Representations of Later Life.* London: Routledge.

Featherstone, M. 1999. Body Modification: An Introduction. *Body & Society*, 5, 1–13.

Featherstone, M. 2007. *Consumer Culture and Postmodernism*. London: Sage Publications.

Featherstone, M. & Wernick, A. 2005. *Images of Aging: Cultural Representations of Later Life*. New York: Routledge.
Fileborn, B., Thorpe, R., Hawkes, G., Minichiello, V. & Pitts, M. 2015. Sex and the (Older) Single Girl: Experiences of Sex and Dating in Later Life. *Journal of Aging Studies*, 33, 67–75.
Fine, M. 2015. Cultures of Care. In: Twigg, J. & Martin, W. (eds) *Routledge Handbook of Cultural Gerontology*. Oxon: Routledge.
Foucault, M. 1976. *The Will to Knowledge: The History of Sexuality Volume 1*. London: Penguin Books.
Foucault, M. 1982. The Subject and Power. *Critical Inquiry*, 8, 777–795.
Foucault, M. 1984a. Nietzsche, Genealogy, History. In: Rabinow, P. (ed.) *The Foucault Reader: An Introduction to Foucault's Thought*. New York: Random House.
Foucault, M. 1984b. Politics and Ethics: An Interview. In: Rabinow, P. (ed.) *The Foucault Reader: An Introduction to Foucault's Thought*. New York: Random House.
Foucault, M. 1990a. *The Care of the Self: The History of Sexuality Volume 3*. London: Penguin Books.
Foucault, M. 1990b. *The Use of Pleasure: The History of Sexuality Volume 2*. USA: Vintage Books.
Foucault, M. 1994. On the Genealogy of Ethics: An Overview of a Work in Progress. In: Rabinow, P. (ed.) *Michel Foucault: Ethics, Subjectivity and Truth*. New York: The New York Press.
Foucault, M. 2005. *The Hermeneutics of the Subject: Lectures at the College De France 1981–1982*. New York: Picador.
Fox, N. 2005. Cultures of Ageing in Thailand and Australia. (What Can an Ageing Body Do?). *Sociology*, 39, 481–498.
Fraser, M. 1997. Feminism, Foucault and Deleuze. *Theory, Culture & Society*, 14, 23–37.
Fraser, S. 2009. Agency Made Over? Cosmetic Surgery and Femininity in Women's Magazines and Makeover Television. In: Heyes, C. & Jones, M. (eds) *Cosmetic Surgery: A Feminist Primer*. Surrey: Ashgate Publishing.
Freeman, E. 2010. *Time Binds: Queer Temporalities, Queer Histories*. Durham: Duke University Press.
Gagne, P. & McGaughey, D. 2002. Designing Women: Cultural Hegemony and the Exercise of Power among Women Who Have Undergone Elective Mammoplasty. *Gender & Society*, 16, 814–838.
Gems, D. 2011. Tragedy and Delight: The Ethics of Decelerated Ageing. *Philosophical Transactions of the Royal Society B: Biological Sciences*, 366, 108–112.
Giddens, A. 1991. *Modernity and Self-identity*. Cambridge: Polity Press.
Gilleard, C. & Higgs, P. 2000. *Cultures of Ageing: Self, Citizen and the Body*. Essex: Prentice Hall.
Gilleard, C. & Higgs, P. 2002. The Third Age: Class, Cohort or Generation? *Ageing & Society*, 22, 369–382.
Gilleard, C. & Higgs, P. 2010. Aging without Agency: Theorizing the Fourth Age. *Aging & Mental Health*, 14, 121–128.
Gilleard, C. & Higgs, P. 2013. *Key Issues in Modern Sociology: Ageing, Corporeality and Embodiment*. London: Anthem Press.
Gilman, S. L. 1999. *Making the Body Beautiful: A Cultural History of Aesthetic Surgery*, New Jersey: Princeton University Press.
Gimlin, D. 2000. Cosmetic Surgery: Beauty as Commodity. *Qualitative Sociology*, 23, 77–98.

Gimlin, D. 2006. The Absent Body Project: Cosmetic Surgery as a Response to Bodily Dys-appearence. *Sociology*, 40, 699–716.
Grey, A. D. N. J. D. 2007. The Natural Biogerontology Portfolio. *Annals of the New York Academy of Sciences*, 1100, 409–423.
Gros, F. 2005. Course Context. In: Gros, F. (ed.) *The Hermeneutics of the Subject: Lectures at the College de France 1981–1982*. New York: Palgrave Macmillian.
Grosz, E. 1994. *Volatile Bodies: Toward a Corporeal Feminism*, Indiana: Allen & Unwin.
Grosz, E. A. 1999. *Becomings: Explorations in Time, Memory, and Futures*, Ithaca, London: Cornell University Press.
Guattari, F. 1995. *Chaosmosis: An Ethico-aesthetic Paradigm*, Sydney: Power Publications.
Gullette, M. 2004. *Aged by Culture*, Chicago: University of Chicago Press.
Hall, S. 1996. Who Needs Identity? In: Hall, S. & Gay, P. D. (eds), *Questions of Cultural Identity*. London: Sage.
Hepworth, M. 2003. Ageing Bodies: Aged by Culture. In: Coupland, J. & Gwyn, R. (eds) *Discourse, the Body and Identity*. Hampshire: Palgrave Macmillan.
Heyes, C. 2007. *Self-transformations: Foucault, Ethics, and Normalised Bodies*. New York: Oxford University Press.
Heyes, C. 2009. All Cosmetic Surgery is 'Ethnic': Asian Eyelids, Feminist Indignation, and the Politics of Whiteness. In: Heyes, C. & Jones, M. (eds) *Cosmetic Surgery: A Feminist Primer*. Surrey: Ashgate Publishing.
Higgs, P. & Gilleard, C. 2014. Frailty, Abjection and the 'Othering' of the Fourth Age. *Health Sociology Review*, 23, 10–19.
Higgs, P., Leontowitsch, M., Stevenson, F. & Rees Jones, I. 2009. Not Just Old and Sick – The 'Will to Health' in Later Life. *Ageing & Society*, 29, 687–707.
Hilário, A. P. 2015. Making Sense of a Changed Physical Body: Why Gender Matters at End of Life. *Journal of Aging Studies*, 33, 58–66.
Hodgetts, D., Chamberlain, K. & Bassett, G. 2003. Between Television and the Audience: Negotiating Representations of Ageing. *Health: An Interdisciplinary Journal for the Social Study of Health, Illness and Medicine*, 7, 417–438.
Hodkinson, P. 2011. Ageing in a Spectacular 'Youth Culture': Continuity, Change and Community amongst Older Goths. *The British Journal of Sociology*, 62, 262.
Hodkinson, P. 2013. Family and Parenthood in an Ageing 'Youth' Culture: A Collective Embrace of Dominant Adulthood? *Sociology*, 47, 1072–1087.
Hulko, W. 2009. The Time- and Context-Contingent Nature of Intersectionality and Interlocking Oppressions. *Affilia*, 24, 44–55.
Hurd Clarke, L. 1999. We're Not Old! Older Women's Negotiation of Aging and Oldness. *Journal of Aging Studies*, 13, 419–440.
Hurd Clarke, L. 2001. Older Women's Bodies and the Self: The Construction of Identity in Later Life. *CRSA/RCSA*, 38, 441–464.
Hurd Clarke, L., Bennett, E. V. & Liu, C. 2014. Aging and Masculinity: Portrayals in Men's Magazines. *Journal of Aging Studies*, 31, 26–33.
Hurd Clarke, L. & Griffin, M. 2007. The Body Natural and the Body Unnatural: Beauty Work and Aging. *Journal of Aging Studies*, 21, 187–201.
Hurd Clarke, L. & Korotchenko, A. 2010. Shades of Grey: To Dye or Not to Dye One's Hair in Later Life. *Ageing & Society*, 30, 1011–1026.
Hurd Clarke, L., Repta, R. & Griffin, M. 2007. Non-Surgical Cosmetic Procedures: Older Women's Perceptions and Experiences. *Journal of Women & Aging*, 19, 69–87.

Jones, M. 2008. *Skintight: An Anatomy of Cosmetic Surgery.* Oxford: Berg.

Katz, S. 1996. *Disciplining Old Age: The Formation of Gerontological Knowlege.* USA: The University Press of Virginia.

Katz, S. 2005. Busy Bodies: Activity, Aging, and the Management of Everyday Life. *Cultural Aging: Life Course, Lifestyle, and Senior Worlds.* Toronto: Broadview Press.

Katz, S. 2015. Ageing, Risk and the Falling Body. In: Twigg, J. & Martin, W. (eds) *Routledge Handbook of Cultural Gerontology.* Oxon: Taylor and Francis.

Katz, S. & Gish, J. 2015. Aging in the Biosocial Order: Repairing Time and Cosmetic Rejuvenation in a Medical Spa Clinic. *Sociological Quarterly,* 56, 40–61.

Katz, S. & Laliberte-Rudman, D. 2005. Exemplars of Retirement: Identity and Agency Between Lifestyle and Social Movement. *Cultural Aging: Life Course, Lifestyle, and Senior Worlds.* Toronto: Broadview Press.

Katz, S. & Marshall, B. 2003. New Sex for Old: Lifestyle, Consumerism, and the Ethics of Aging Well. *Journal of Aging Studies,* 17, 3–16.

Kontos, P. 2015. Dementia and Embodiment. In: Twigg, J. & Martin, W. (eds) *Routledge Handbook of Cultural Gerontology.* Oxon: Routledge.

Koutsogeorgou, E., Davies, J. K., Aranda, K., Zissi, A., Chatzikou, M., Cerniauskaite, M., Quintas, R., Raggi, A. & Leonardi, M. 2014. Healthy and Active Ageing: Social Capital in Health Promotion. *Health Education Journal,* 73, 627–641.

Krainitzki, E. 2014. Judi Dench's Age-inappropriateness and the Role of M: Challenging Normative Temporality. *Journal of Aging Studies,* 29, 32.

Laliberte Rudman, D. L. 2006. Shaping the Active, Autonomous and Responsible Modern Retiree: An Analysis of Discursive Technologies and their Links with Neo-liberal Political Rationality. *Ageing & Society,* 26, 181–201.

Lester, R. J. 1997. The (Dis)embodied Self in Anorexia Nervosa. *Social Science and Medicine,* 44, 479–489.

Lodge, A. C. & Umberson, D. 2013. Age and Embodied Masculinities: Midlife Gay and Heterosexual Men Talk about their Bodies. *Journal of Aging Studies,* 27, 225–232.

Longino, C. F. & Powell, J. L. 2004. Embodiment and the Study of Aging. In: Berdayes, V., Esposito, L. & Murphy, J. W. (eds) *The Body in Human Inquiry: Interdisciplinary Explorations of Embodiment.* New Jersey: Hampton Press.

Marshall, B. L. & Rahman, M. 2015. Celebrity, Ageing and the Construction of 'Third Age' Identities. *International Journal of Cultural Studies,* 18, 577–593.

Mendes, F. R. 2013. Active Ageing: A Right or a Duty? *Health Sociology Review,* 22, 174–185.

Montemurro, B. & Siefken, J. M. 2014. Cougars on the Prowl? New Perceptions of Older Women's Sexuality. *Journal of Aging Studies,* 28, 35–43.

Morgan, K. P. 2009. Women and the Knife: Cosmetic Surgery and the Colonization of Women's Bodies. In: Heyes, C. & Jones, M. (eds) *Cosmetic Surgery: A Feminist Primer.* Surrey: Ashgate Publishing.

Moulaert, T. & Biggs, S. 2013. International and European Policy on Work and Retirement: Reinventing Critical Perspectives on Active Ageing and Mature Subjectivity. *Human Relations,* 66, 23–43.

Öberg, P. 2003. Image versus Experience of the Aging Body. In: Faircloth, C. A. (ed.) *Aging Bodies: Images and Everyday Experience.* Walnut Creek: AltMira Press.

Paulson, S. & Willig, C. 2008. Older Women and Everyday Talk about the Ageing Body. *Journal of Health Psychology,* 13, 106–120.

Phillipson, C. 2013. *Ageing*. 1 ed. Hoboken: Wiley.

Phoenix, C. & Smith, B. 2011. Telling a (Good?) Counterstory of Aging: Natural Bodybuilding Meets the Narrative of Decline. *Journals of Gerontology Series B: Psychological Sciences and Social Sciences*, 66B, 628–639.

Pitts-Taylor, V. 2007. *Surgery Junkies: Wellness and Pathology in Cosmetic Culture*. New Jersey: Rutgers University Press.

Pitts-Taylor, V. 2009. Becoming/Being a Cosmetic Surgery Patient: Semantic Instability and the Intersubjective Self. *Studies in Gender and Sexuality*, 10, 119–128.

Pitts, V. 2003. *In the Flesh: The Cultural Politics of Body Modification*. New York: *Palgrave Macmillan*.

Pitts, V. 1999. Body Modification, Self-Mutilation and Agency in Media Accounts of a Subculture. *Body & Society*, 5, 291–303.

Powell, J. L. 2006. *Social Theory and Aging*. USA: Rowman & Littlefield Publishers.

Powell, J. L. 2011. *Aging and Social Policy: A Foucauldian Excursion*. New York: Nova Science Publishers.

Powell, J. L. & Biggs, S. 2000. Managing Old Age: The Disciplinary Web of Power, Surveillance and Normalization. *Journal of Aging and Identity*, 5, 3–13.

Probyn, E. 1993. *Sexing the Self: Gendered Positions in Cultural Studies*. London: Routledge.

Quéniart, A. & Charpentier, M. 2012. Older Women and their Representations of Old Age: A Qualitative Analysis. *Ageing and Society*, 32, 983–1007.

Rabinow, P. (ed.) 1984. *The Foucault Reader: An Introduction to Foucault's Thought*. New York: Random House.

Riach, K., Rumens, N. & Tyler, M. 2014. Un/doing Chrononormativity: Negotiating Ageing, Gender and Sexuality in Organizational Life. *Organization Studies*, 35, 1677–1698.

Rose, N. 2001. The Politics of Life Itself. *Theory, Culture & Society*, 18, 1–30.

Rowntree, M. R. 2014. 'Comfortable in My Own Skin': A New Form of Sexual Freedom for Ageing Baby Boomers. *Journal of Aging Studies*, 31, 150–158.

Ryan, D. 2001. Adding Years Gracefully. *The Age*.

Sánchez Palacios, C., Trianes Torres, M. V. & Blanca Mena, M. J. 2009. Negative Aging Stereotypes and their Relation with Psychosocial Variables in the Elderly Population. *Archives of Gerontology & Geriatrics*, 48, 385–390.

Sedgwick, E. K. 1997. Paranoid Reading and Reparative Reading; or, You're So Paranoid, You probably Think this Introduction Is about You. In: Sedgwick, E. K. (ed.) *Novel Gazing: Queer Readings in Fiction*. London: Duke University Press.

Shilling, C. 2003. *The Body and Social Theory*. London: Sage Publications.

Slevin, K. 2010. 'If I Had Lots of Money… I'd Have a Body Makeover': Managing the Aging Body. *Social Forces*, 88, 1003–1020.

Smith, F., Wainwright, E., Buckingham, S. & Marandet, E. 2011. Women, Work–Life Balance and Quality of Life: Case Studies from the United Kingdom and Republic of Ireland. *Gender, Place & Culture*, 18, 603–610.

Sullivan, N. 2001. *Tattooed Bodies: Subjectivity, Textuality, Ethics, and Pleasure*. USA: Praeger Publishers.

The Canadian Press. 2002. More People 65 and Older Getting Cosmetic Surgery. 24 July.

Thomas, R., Hardy, C., Cutcher, L. & Ainsworth, S. 2014. What's Age Got to Do with It? On the Critical Analysis of Age and Organizations. *Organization Studies*, 35, 1569–1584.

Tulle-Winton, E. 2000. Old Bodies. In: Hancock, P., Hughes, B., Jagger, E., Paterson, K., Russell, R., Tulle-Winton, E. & Tyler, M. (eds) *The Body, Culture and Society: An Introduction*. Buckingham: Open University Press.

Tulle, E. 2008a. Acting your Age? Sports Science and the Ageing Body. *Journal of Aging Studies*, 22, 340–347.

Tulle, E. 2008b. The Ageing Body and the Ontology of Ageing: Athletic Competence in Later Life. *Body & Society*, 14, 1–19.

Turner, B. S. 1991. Recent Developments in the Theory of the Body. In: Featherstone, M., Hepworth, M. & Turner, B. S. (eds) *The Body: Social Process and Cultural Theory*. London: Sage Publications.

Twigg, J. 2004. The Body, Gender, and Age: Feminist Insights in Social Gerontology. *Journal of Aging Studies*, 18, 59–73.

Twigg, J. 2010. Clothing and Dementia: A Neglected Dimension? *Journal of Aging Studies*, 24, 223–230.

Twigg, J. 2012. Adjusting the Cut: Fashion, the Body and Age on the UK High Street. *Ageing and Society*, 32, 1030–1054.

Twigg, J. & Majima, S. 2014. Consumption and the Constitution of Age: Expenditure Patterns on Clothing, Hair and Cosmetics among Post-war 'Baby Boomers'. *Journal of Aging Studies*, 30, 23–32.

Twigg, J. & Martin, W. (eds) 2015. *Routledge International Handbooks: Routledge Handbook of Cultural Gerontology*. Oxon & New York: Taylor and Francis.

Valentine, G. 2007. Theorizing and Researching Intersectionality: A Challenge for Feminist Geography. *Professional Geographer*, 59, 10–21.

Van Dyk, S. 2014. The Appraisal of Difference: Critical Gerontology and the Active-ageing Paradigm. *Journal of Aging Studies*, 31, 93–103.

Villa, P. 2011. Embodiment is Always More: Intersectionality, Subjection and the Body. In: Lutz, H., Vivar, M. T. H. & Supik, L. (eds) *Framing Intersectionality: Debates on a Multi-faceted Concept in Gender Studies*. London: Ashgate Publishing.

Wada, M., Hurd Clarke, L. & Rozanova, J. 2015. Constructions of Sexuality in Later Life: Analyses of Canadian Magazine and Newspaper Portrayals of Online Dating. *Journal of Aging Studies*, 32, 40–49.

Wahidin, A. & Powell, J. L. 2003. Reconfiguring Old Bodies: From the Biomedical Model to a Critical Epistemology. *Sincronia*.

Ward, R., Campbell, S. & Keady, J. 2014. 'Once I had money in my pocket, I was every colour under the sun': Using 'Appearance Biographies' to Explore the Meanings of Appearance for People with Dementia. *Journal of Aging Studies*, 30, 64–72.

Warren, C. A. B. 1998. Aging and Identity in Premodern Times. *Research on Aging*, 20, 11–35.

WHO. 2015. *Active Ageing: A Policy Framework* [Online]. Available: http://www.who.int/ageing/active_ageing/en/ [Accessed 12 August 2015].

Wolf, N. 1990. *The Beauty Myth: How Images of Beauty Are Used Against Women*. London: Chatto & Windus.

Yuval-Davis, N. 2006. Intersectionality and Feminist Politics. *European Journal of Women's Studies*, 13, 193–209.

Ziegler, F. 2012. 'You have to engage with life, or life will go away': An Intersectional Life Course Analysis of Older Women's Social Participation in a Disadvantaged Urban Area. *Geoforum*, 43, 1296–1305.

2 *Designing* 'older' rather than denying ageing

Introduction

Discourses of ageing, anti-ageing and ageism shape a multiplicity of accounts on the rising trend of older people undergoing cosmetic surgery in the international mass media. There are those that position cosmetic surgery within the 'pursuit of eternal youth', 'fear of ageing' and wanting to 'deny that we are getting old' (Ryan, 2001). These buttress well with those that charge cosmetic surgery and its adherents with complicity in societal ageism or 'a collective social prejudice against getting old and being old' (Stock, 1996). And, then there are accounts of 'the latest generation of pensioners as "the new old" who are determined to combat the ageing process by buying youthful brands, adventure holidays and cosmetic surgery' (N.A., 2005). These latter accounts seem to suggest a radical refusal of ageing and resistance of old age through 'youthful' pursuits. Across these media accounts, ideas about whether ageing is being 'denied' or 'combatted' give rise to ethical concerns framed by a dichotomy in which cosmetic surgery is rendered either an oppressive or liberating practice. Whilst apparently polarized, both accounts reinscribe the 'ageing' of the body into the problematization of older people and cosmetic surgery. The dichotomy that underpins these media standpoints mirrors positions on structure and agency within feminist and critical ageing studies scholarship on cosmetic surgery (see Chapter 1). Rather than reproducing these positions in relation to ageing, this chapter provides an approach to understanding cosmetic surgery as a practice that is shaped by norms *and* provides possibilities for agency. This is strategically important for the cultural politics of 'older' because it provides an opportunity for new insights into the cultural spaces in which *becoming* 'older' is possible and the ways in which cosmetic surgery is being appropriated to this task.

The depth of engagement offered here in terms of developing such an approach is ethically important. Much research in the human and social sciences assumes ethical neutrality as if, in Rabinow's (2003: 8) terms, 'the reception of objective truth had no necessary consequences for the ethical state of the subject who received it'. Critical of this ethical blind spot, Rabinow (2003: 2) states:

> The currently reigning modes of research in the human sciences are, it seems to me, deficient in vital aspects. Those deficiencies are especially marked in the strained relations between an ever-accumulating body of information, the ways that information is given narrative and conceptual form, and how this knowledge fits into a conduct of life.

To examine how knowledge 'fits into a conduct of life' for older people, requires an approach based on a dynamic nexus between theory and empirical data. In this approach, theory is put to work following Foucault's (1984: 88) assertion that 'knowledge is not meant for understanding; it is made for cutting'. It will become clear that this understanding of the use of theory elegantly synchronizes with cosmetic surgery as a practice for enacting a 'cutting critique'. The task of 'cutting' to which theory is charged, involves 'rupturing' interpretations of cosmetic surgery undertaken by 'older' people as denying ageing through a problematization of 'truth'. As Foucault (1994c: 275) suggests: 'interpretation does not clarify a matter to be interpreted, which offers itself passively; it can only seize, and violently, an already-present interpretation, which it must overthrow, upset, shatter with the blows of a hammer'.

Amid the shards of already present interpretations, a cultural space will emerge in which it becomes possible to 'think differently' (Foucault, 1990b: 9). The empirical data provides the contemporary discourses that enliven the theory and put it to work to speak to the present. As a practice of body modification, cosmetic surgery is significant because the body is the nexus or site where 'forces of cultural reproduction, social structuration, and reflexivity' intersect to constitute the 'self' (Gabardi, 2001: 88). This cultural richness and complexity requires a nuanced reading, one that 'is necessarily beyond the stability of a humanist identity' and 'grounded in a politics marked by selves and...inspired and engaged with the subjectivities enmeshed within our everyday lives' (Probyn, 1993: 109). Thus, what is needed, are ways to explore how 'older' people engage cultural practices to navigate, adapt or adopt cultural positions and thus constitute their subjective experience of 'older'. Theoretical accounts and cultural texts and practices therefore need to be interpreted and possibly rearticulated through subjective accounts of experience by 'older people'. Such an approach enables exploration of how culture relates to subjectivity, identity or lived experiences of selfhood. Following Twigg (2004: 62), this approach 'recognizes that personal struggles and experiences offer an important touchstone for academic theorizing', one that is 'grounded in the voices of those who are themselves subject to' constitution as 'older'.

Foucault's thought on the subject

To begin thinking through Foucault's writing on ethics in terms of how cosmetic surgery might be implicated in processes of *becoming* 'older', an introduction and overview of Foucault's thought on the subject will prove useful. Neither strictly a philosopher nor historian, Foucault shaped an interdisciplinary space at the intersection of both disciplines that he described as the History of Systems of Thought. Beginning with a question posed in the present concerning contemporary forms of subjective experience, including madness (Foucault, 1961), delinquency (Foucault, 1991a) and sexuality (Foucault, 1976, 1990b, 1990a), Foucault analysed historical texts to examine the ways in which subjective experience is constituted and undergoes modification in thought. He states, 'There is no experience that is not a way of thinking and cannot be analysed from the viewpoint of a history of thought' (Foucault, 1994e: 201). Toward the end of his career, Foucault (1990b) conceptualized his analyses as having been elaborated along three interrelated axes – truth (fields of knowledge), power (types of normativity) and the subject (forms of subjectivity). What counts as truth, according to Foucault, is an effect of rules for the production of legitimate knowledge and he referred to these rules as 'games of truth' and the knowledge legitimated by these rules as 'regimens of truth' (Foucault, 1981: 133; Foucault, 1994a). Commenting on his body of scholarship, Foucault places his concern with games of truth as central to understanding how the human subject is defined. He writes:

> I have tried to discover how the human subject entered into games of truth, whether they be games of truth which take on the form of science or which refer to a scientific model, or games of truth like those that can be found in institutions or practices of control…I've tried to show how, in scientific creation, the human subject will be defined as an individual who talks, who works, who lives.
>
> (Foucault, 1994a: 1)

What Foucault suggests is that, as an object of scientific knowledges, the human subject is productively constituted through regimens of power. This intimate dynamic connecting power and knowledge was referred to by Foucault as power/knowledge and he analysed this nexus through discourse.

Foucault (1972: 49) conceptualized discourse as 'practices that systematically form the objects of which they speak'. In his analyses, Foucault (1972: 47–48 emphasis in original) sought to define objects: 'without reference to the *ground*, the *foundation of things*, but by relating them to the body of rules that enable them to form as objects of a discourse and thus constitute the conditions of their historical existence'.

Foucault's (1972: 49) use of the term 'discourse' does not refer to a 'mere intersection of things and words', between reality and language, where language is used to designate objects or 'things'. Rather, he suggests 'Discourses should be understood as statements with a material existence' (Foucault, 2005: 322). As Hook (2001: 524) elaborates, 'Foucault's conception of discourse is situated far more closely to knowledge, materiality and power than it is to language'.

In Foucault's early writing, he analysed the subject as 'the objective product of systems of knowledge and power' (Gros, 2005: 513). These analyses, which presented a figure of the subject as passively inscribed by relations of power/knowledge, radically challenged the essentialism of the humanistic and phenomenological subject.[1] His emphasis on the axes of knowledge and power continues up until the first volume of the *History of Sexuality*, in which he establishes a focus upon 'the relations of power that contribute to the constitution of the desiring subject via its insertion into domains of knowledge and normative schemes' (Fillion, 2005: 50). In this volume, Foucault presents a methodological framework for the analysis of power and provides a chronological and thematic schema for the following volumes. However, as Gros (2005: 508) remarks, 'None of these books ever appeared'. After eight years, volumes two and three of the *History of Sexuality* were published simultaneously and constituted a 'major recasting' (Rabinow, 1994: xvii) of Foucault's project in terms of the analytic focus and historical period that provides the substantive texts for analysis.

In volumes two and three of the *History of Sexuality*, Foucault is concerned with desire as an ethical problem and tracing historical modifications to the ethical domain in relation to sexuality. However, in these books Foucault orients his analyses according to his third axis – forms of subjectivity – in order to examine 'the constitution of the subject as an object for himself' (Florence, 1994: 461). For some of his interlocutors, this move was interpreted as radically undermining his earlier position regarding the essentialism of the phenomenological and humanist subject (see for example, Paras, 2006). In his own commentary however, Foucault (Florence, 1994: 461) regards this shift as complementing his prior analyses of the 'modes according to which the subject was able to be inserted as an object in the games of truth'. Rather than recourse to a pre-discursive subject, Foucault sought to determine how the ethical subject was constituted through an elaboration of a form of relation to self in which 'the subject experiences himself in a regimen of truth where he relates to himself' (Florence, 1994: 461). Foucault illustrates how the elaboration of this reflexive relation of the self to itself was enacted through practices of self. In *Subjectivity and Truth*, he defines practices of the self as:

> the procedures, which no doubt exist in every civilization, offered or prescribed to individuals in order to determine their identity, maintain it, or transform it in terms of a certain number of ends, through relations of self- mastery or self knowledge.
>
> (Foucault, 1994g: 87)

What Foucault was arguing, is that the available practices of self in society and culture precondition the formation of the subject by providing modes of subjectivation.[2]

The historical-cultural framework in which Foucault located his analyses was not Western Modernity, but rather Greco-Roman Antiquity. As Foucault (1994e: 204) explains:

> I found myself spanning eras in a way that took me farther and farther from the chronological outline I had first decided on, both in order to address myself to periods when the effect of scientific knowledges and the complexity of normative systems were less, and in order eventually to make out the forms of relation to the self different from those characterizing the [modern] experience of sexuality.

As this quotation suggests, the significance of this historical period for Foucault was that it enabled him to reveal alternative forms of relation to the self. What Foucault discovered during this historical period was an 'aesthetic' form of relationship between the subject and ethical principles. As Foucault (1990b: 92) writes: 'classical antiquity's moral reflection concerning the pleasures was not directed towards a codification of acts, nor a hermeneutics of the subject, but towards a stylization of attitudes and an aesthetics of existence'.

What Foucault (1994d: 230) suggests is that the principal target of this kind of ethics was 'a problem of personal choice' rather than a 'hermeneutics of the self' that establishes 'truth' as an essential nature of being. In this ethical domain, practices of self were 'intentional and voluntary actions' enmeshed with 'rules of conduct' engaged to transform the self into an ethical subject whose life 'carries certain aesthetic values and meets certain stylistic criteria' (Foucault, 1990b: 10–11). Practices of self therefore imply a creative self-fashioning of the subject to achieve a desirable mode of being. Foucault contrasts this aesthetic and freely chosen ethic with the universal, quasi-juridical morality of Christianity and demonstrates how through certain modifications 'in the first centuries of our era, an obligation to tell the truth about oneself was established' (Gros, 2005: 510).

Despite proclaiming his apparent enthusiasm for ethics as aesthetics with the rhetorical question, 'Couldn't everyone's life become a work of art?' (Foucault, 1994d: 236), Foucault was not advocating a 'return' to ancient Greek and Roman ethics. These, he argued, arose in an entirely different context. When asked in an interview with Dreyfus and Rabinow (1982: 231) whether the 'Greeks offer an attractive and plausible alternative', Foucault responds 'No! I am not looking for an alternative; you can't find the solution of a problem in the solution of another problem raised at another moment by other people'. Rather than unequivocally advocating ancient ethics, Foucault suggests the possibility of unrealized alternatives for the present (Rabinow, 1994). Specifically, as Fillion (2005: 56, emphasis in original) argues, it is in 'Foucault's insistence on *ethics* and the practices that constitute them as a contrast with *morality* and the codes or prescriptions it seeks to instantiate, that many see the possibility for a new ethos within our late-modern condition'.

Foucault's thought on practices of the self as constitutive of the ethical subject in relation to an aesthetics of existence thus provides an approach for thinking about an ethic of 'older' in which cosmetic surgery is engaged in the creative self-fashioning of 'older' rather than denying age or ageing. To explore how this aesthetic ethic of the self materializes in the social and cultural discourses that constitute the contemporary ethical domain, the chapter turns to the ethical principles that Foucault described in his historical work and considers these in relation to advanced neoliberal consumer society.

Twin ethical principles: 'Know yourself' and 'care of the self'

According to Foucault (2005: 69), 'know yourself' and 'care of self' constitute twin ethical principles that rival for dominance in a 'dynamic entanglement' in models of ethics, or more specifically ethical subjectivity, in philosophical thought. As Davidson (2005: xxi) points out in his introduction to *The Hermeneutics of the Subject*, the relations between these principles form the 'axis for understanding the historically and philosophically modifiable connection between the subject and truth'. In Greek and Roman antiquity, practices of ethical self formation were primarily organized and given meaning by the principle of 'care of the self' which 'supported an extremely rich and dense set of notions, practices, ways of being, forms of existence, and so on' (Foucault, 2005: 12). Taking care of one's self meant 'working on' or 'being concerned with' the self by engaging in ethical practices geared towards achieving an existence characterized by virtue and beauty (Foucault, 1994d). This work on the self was not an obligation imposed on the individual but rather a mode of subjectivation characterized by aesthetic and ethical principles and associated with an active freedom. During Greek and Roman antiquity, Foucault (1994b: 284) writes, 'the care of the self was the mode in which individual freedom – or civic liberty, up to a point – was reflected [*se réfléchie*] as an ethics'.

During Greek antiquity, 'know yourself' was framed through 'care of self' in that knowledge of the self was required in order to take care of the self. As Foucault (2005: 82) suggests, in this ethical domain, 'To take care of the self is to know oneself'. Taking care of oneself thus required a relationship to knowledge but not in the sense of a requirement to decipher the truth of an inner essence. Rather, it meant being 'equipped' and able to act appropriately in relation to moral precepts. In *The Use of Pleasure*, Foucault (1990b: 89) writes:

> The relation to truth was a structural, instrumental, and ontological condition for establishing the individual as a moderate subject leading a life of moderation; it was not an epistemological condition enabling the individual to recognize himself in his singularity as a desiring subject.

Foucault contrasted this Greco-Roman relation between the subject and truth with the modern 'hermeneutic' model to suggest that 'knowledge of the world is a relevant part of the subject's practice on himself' however, this 'does not involve the subject becoming the object of a true discourse' (Foucault, 2005: 243). What Foucault's analyses of Greco- Roman texts suggest, is that 'care of the self' opened into a stylization of attitudes and aesthetics of existence rather than an essentialist subject. The significance of this analytic insight was to suggest the possibility of an alternative relationship between the subject and truth to that founded within Christianity and Western modernity.

In *The Care of the Self*, Foucault (1990a) suggests that through certain modifications, the mode of subjectivation associated with the famous Delphic prescription 'know yourself' came to dominate and to some extent subsume 'care of self' so that in Western thought and ethics, 'care of self' was 'left in the shadow' (Foucault, 2005: 12). Foucault identifies the 'Cartesian moment' associated with the Enlightenment as the historical point at which 'know yourself' was philosophically requalified by discrediting 'care of the self' (Foucault, 2005: 14). With the establishment of rationalism, 'truth' was made self-evident and games of truth were underpinned by objectivity to constitute the scientific method. What this meant was that the ethical subject was no longer required to transform the self to obtain access to 'truth'. Foucault (2005) suggests that this disconnected epistemology from spirituality. And hence, with this 'Cartesian moment' the 'modern age of the relations between the subject and truth' began (Davidson, 2005: xxiv).

Within Christian ethics, 'care of the self' became problematic and the principle 'know yourself' firmly took hold to establish the truth of an individual's being as the foundation for ethical practice. 'This new Christian self', Foucault (1994d: 274) writes, 'had to be constantly examined because in this self were lodged concupiscence and desires of the flesh. From that moment on, the self was no longer something to be made but something to be renounced and deciphered'.

In this Christian mode of subjection, self-decipherment was a requirement for renouncing the self. Foucault understood confessional practices as central to this decipherment and integral to the production of the subject. By speaking the 'truth' of the self, the true self was revealed and could be renounced. Over time the Christian practices of self-examination and confession extended into secular practices of the self, particularly through the development of psychology and psychoanalysis, to provide the basis for contemporary ethics and modern hermeneutics of the subject.

During a lecture in the course *The Hermeneutics of the Subject*, Foucault (2005: 12) suggests that there 'is clearly something a bit disturbing for us in this principle of care of the self'. He goes on to talk about how notions of 'taking care of the self', 'looking after' oneself or 'devoting oneself to oneself' have taken on negative meanings. These negative meanings he suggests, have their basis in several traditions of moral thought to which 'care of self' sounds like a 'desire for radical ethical change, a sort of moral dandyism'[3] (Foucault, 2005: 12). Through these traditions of moral thought, 'care of the self' has become associated with individualistic and superficial notions of self-absorption, narcissism and vanity. When asked in an interview, conducted in 1983 with Dreyfus and Rabinow, whether the Greek concern with the self is an early version of contemporary self-absorption, however, Foucault makes this point clear:

> In the Californian cult of the self, one is supposed to discover one's true self, to separate it from that which might obscure or alienate it, to decipher its truth thanks to psychological or psychoanalytic science, which is supposed to be able to tell you what your true self is. Therefore, not only do I not identify this ancient culture of the self with what you might call the Californian cult of the self, I think they are diametrically opposed.
>
> (Foucault, 1994d: 271)

As this quotation suggests, the 'cult of the self' that was apparent to Foucault in California, was based in a hermeneutics of the subject rather than an aesthetic mode of ethical stylization such as that which characterized the ancient Greek 'culture of the self'.

As Foucault's analyses demonstrate, the contemporary Western mode of Cartesian ethics is only one possibility, one that is historically situated and entirely different to the relation between subject and truth in ancient Greek and Roman ethics. Whilst 'know yourself' has dominated the ethical domain since the time of the Enlightenment, Foucault's insistence on surfacing its twin principle 'care of the self' exhorts us to explore how this principle may also operate in contemporary contexts. Given Foucault's death in 1984 we will never know how he would perceive the current ethical climate in advanced neoliberal consumer societies. In an interview held shortly before his death, however, Foucault (1988a: 49) states that his interest in Antiquity was because:

> for a whole series of reasons, the idea of a morality as obedience to a code of rules is now disappearing, has already disappeared. And to this absence of morality corresponds, must correspond, the search for an aesthetics of existence.

This raises the question as to whether contemporary consumer culture that produces an 'aestheticization of everyday life' may be understood in terms of a transformation in the relations between care of the self and knowledge of the self to constitute a new formation of aesthetic ethics.

Contemporary 'ethopolitics': a nexus between neoliberal politics and consumer culture

In social conditions characterized as 'liquid' (Bauman, 2008), consumer culture and the neoliberal political economy together provide the conditions of possibility for the 'aestheticization of everyday life' and surface of emergence for contemporary discourses shaping 'older' subjectivities (see Chapter 1). At present, neoliberalism is the dominant political rationality and ethos of government in Western democratic societies. Political scholars Barry, Osborne and Rose (1996: 10) explain that neoliberal political reason has involved the 'invention and/or deployment of a whole array of organizational forms and technical methods in order to extend the field within which a certain kind of economic freedom might be practiced in the form of personal autonomy, enterprise and choice'. As a political rationality, neoliberalism is premised upon individual freedom and the strategic insight that 'power works most effectively when it works through shaping the way in which individuals enact their freedom' (Rose, n.d.). In neoliberal societies, economic choice is the means by which individuals are governed according to the shaping of possibilities through which to enact their freedom (Hamann, 2009: 38). Such an approach involves governing 'at a distance' through the constitution of the neoliberal subject as a self-governing, autonomous, enterprising consumer (Rose, 2007).

The expansion of the field in which market-based rationalities operate through neoliberal policies has meant that individuals are increasingly positioned as 'consumers' in a greater diversity of social spheres including 'traditional social goods such as healthcare, welfare, and social security' (Hamann, 2009: 40). The colonization of neoliberal rationality across so many spheres of life constitutes, what some social and cultural theorists consider to be, 'The Consumer Society' (Baudrillard, 1998; Bauman, 2007). That consumerism is an attribute of such societies means that it has become:

> the principal propelling and operating force of society, a force that coordinates systemic reproduction, social integration, social stratification and the formation of human individuals, as well as playing a major role in the processes of individual and group self-identification and in the selection and pursuit of individual life policies.
>
> (Bauman, 2007: 28)

The freedom to select and pursue individual life policies through consumer choice requires consumers to act as morally responsible agents in the conduct of life. What this means is that, through neoliberal policies and consumer practices, 'Exploitation, domination, and every other form of social inequality is rendered invisible as social phenomenon to the extent that each individual's social condition is judged as nothing other than the effect of his or her own choices and investments' (Hamann, 2009: 43). Individual consumer health, wealth and happiness are positioned as the products of freely made choices during the life course whilst a 'mismanaged life' is attributed 'to the moral failure of that individual' (Hamann, 2009: 44).

Through the promotion of health, financial independence and happiness, neoliberal governmental imperatives to reduce State dependence, and thus expenditure, align with individual ethics of a life well lived. Rose (2007: 27) refers to this nexus as 'ethopolitics', which he defines as those 'attempts to shape the conduct of human beings by acting upon their sentiments, beliefs, and values – in short by acting on ethics'. He goes on to elaborate:

> In the politics of our present, notably in the revival of communitarian themes, the ethos of human existence – the sentiments, moral nature, or

> guiding beliefs of persons, groups, or institutions – has come to provide the "medium" within which the self-government of the autonomous individual can be connected up with the imperatives of good government…"ethopolitics" concerns itself with the self-techniques by which human beings should judge and act upon themselves to make themselves better than they are.

In this ethopolitical context, where the burden of responsibility for social welfare is shouldered by the self-governing individual, assessment, prevention and management of risk through an expansive and expanding focus on 'lifestyle' is a governmental task. Supporting individuals to make the 'right lifestyle choices' are a framework of scientific knowledge and increasing array of expert advisors including, therapists, counsellors, life coaches, wealth management advisors, nutritionists, personal fitness trainers, and 'self-help' technologies. These 'experts' provide an authoritative discourse to 'infuse lifestyle with rational techniques and imperatives and thereby project a new configuration of subjectivity and social power' (Binkley, 2007: 117). These discourses provide the *tekhne* or 'know how' (Foucault, 2005) concerning the practices in which the ethical subject must engage to attain health and wellbeing.

Self-fashioning a 'lifestyle' within consumer culture takes on an ethical dimension associated with virtues in the context of, what Featherstone (2007), among others, refers to as the 'aestheticization of everyday life'. Featherstone (2007: 65) suggests that in one sense 'the aestheticization of everyday life can refer to the project of turning life into a work of art' and that the virtues associated with doing so mean that 'the aesthetic life is the ethically good life' (Featherstone, 2007: 47). As a feature of the present:

> a life of aesthetic consumption and the need to form life into an aesthetically pleasing whole…should be related to the development of mass consumption in general and the pursuit of new tastes and sensations and the construction of distinctive lifestyles which has become central to consumer culture.
>
> (Featherstone, 2007: 66)

As this quotation suggests, in consumer society and culture, individuals come to stylize their lives through practices of consumption to create a 'lifestyle'. The lifestyle fashioned by an individual is thus an outward and visible manifestation of 'individuality, self- expression, and a stylistic self-consciousness' (Featherstone, 2007: 81).

In his theorization of consumption, Bauman (2007: 15, emphasis in original) suggests that, 'Consumer's "subjectivity" is made out of shopping choices… what is assumed to be the *materialization* of the inner truth of the self is in fact an *idealization* of the material – objectified – traces of consumer choices'. What Bauman is suggesting, is that shopping choices do not reflect an inner truth, but rather, constitute the subject in particular ways. He suggests that

'To complete the popular, revised version of Descarte's Cogito, "I shop therefore I am…", "a subject" could and should be added' (Bauman, 2007: 17). The 'traces of consumer choices' that Bauman refers to suggest the operation of a system of signification. Baudrillard (1998) for instance, states that alongside functionality, commodities possess value in terms of what they signify such as prestige or good taste. For Bauman and Baudrillard, commodities are consumed to signify something about the consumer and practices of consumption constitute our subjectivity. The force compelling the consumer to purchase commodities for what they signify is therefore not need but desire. The freedom to desire and choose what is desirable within a system of signification enables consumers to stylize an identity. The significance of this discussion of the self as a lifestyle project is that rather than based on scientific knowledge or 'truth', consumer practices constitute the subject through 'an ethics of the "aesthetics of existence"' (Besley and Peters, 2007: 41).

Rose (2001) observes that in neoliberal consumer culture, selfhood has become intrinsically somatic and ethical practices increasingly take the body as a key site for work on the self. As a feature of our present, he writes about 'somatic ethics' which he explains are 'ethics not in the sense of moral principles' but rather 'the values for the conduct of a life – that accords a central place to corporeal, bodily existence' (Rose, 2007: 6). Prior to Rose's work, Baudrillard (1998: 129) argued that 'the body has today become an object of salvation' and has 'literally taken over that moral and ideological function from the soul'. This contemporary ethical domain in Western societies compels individuals '*to put themselves in the service of their own bodies*' because 'one has a duty to take care of oneself' (Baudrillard, 1998: 140, emphasis as original). In the contemporary ethical domain, taking care of the body has thus become synonymous with taking care of the self, and practices for cultivating the body operate in the context of virtues belonging to an art of living. In this context, cosmetic surgery might be understood as a practice of self-care engaged to stylize 'older' subjectivities. To pursue this further, in terms of how the process of *becoming* older can be analysed in relation to cosmetic surgery and this ethopolitical context, I return to Foucault's work which provides a theoretical approach to understanding the formation of the embodied ethical subject.

Becoming: the formation of the embodied ethical subject

In Foucault's work, questions of the body are fundamental to his analyses of how knowledge and power constitute the subject. Foucault (1984: 83) argues that the materiality of the body is the 'locus of a dissociated self (adopting the illusion of a substantial unity)'. He suggests that through the investment of power in the body the 'interiority' of the subject is produced:

> Rather than seeing this soul as the reactivated remnants of an ideology, one would see it as the present correlative of a certain technology of

> power over the body…it is produced permanently around, on, within the body by the functioning of a power that is exercised on those punished – and, in a more general way, on those one supervises, trains and corrects.
> (Foucault, 1991a: 29)

What Foucault is suggesting here, is that the 'soul' or 'self' is an effect of power acting upon, and being enfolded into, the body. He goes on to state that on this foundation of the 'soul' a whole corpus of discursive concepts relating to this interiority have been assembled, including 'psyche, subjectivity, personality, consciousness etc.' (Foucault, 1991a: 29–30). These concepts emerge from the human and social sciences and form the basis for 'the moral claims of humanism' (Foucault, 1991a: 29–30).

Foucault's theorization of subjectivation is elaborated in his texts on ethics and particularly the second volume of *The History of Sexuality*. In this text, Foucault (1990b: 26) differentiates between moral codes and ethical practices stating:

> a rule of conduct is one thing; the conduct that may be measured by this rule is another. But another thing still is the manner in which one ought to "conduct oneself" – that is, the manner in which one ought to form oneself as an ethical subject acting in reference to the prescriptive elements that make up the code.

In his analyses Foucault (1990b: 26, 30) focuses on ethics, or 'how one ought to form oneself as an ethical subject' and 'the exercises by which he makes of himself an object to be known, and on the practices that enable him to transform his own mode of being'. For Foucault, ethics is concerned with the relation of self to self, established through exercises of self-reflection, self-examination, self-decipherment, self-transformation and so on. This reflexive relationship is what constitutes subjectivities. Drawing on his reading of Foucault's theorization of subjectivation, Deleuze (1986: 100) suggests that subjectivity can be thought of as a fold. He writes, 'it is as if the outside folded back to create a doubling, allow a relation to oneself to emerge, and constitute an inside which is hollowed out and develops its own dimension'. Similarly, Butler (1997: 6) describes the folding of force as a 'twisting' that constitutes the subject's self-identity and asserts that 'the subject is the effect of power in recoil'.

The substantive texts for Foucault's analyses of ethics came from Greco-Roman antiquity because they revealed the formation of subjectivity without recourse to a hermeneutics of the subject. Through his historical analyses, Foucault sought to trace how, through certain modifications to the ethical domain, the contemporary mode of ethics emerged from those of antiquity. This book does not present historical research but rather is concerned with analysing the contemporary ethical domain in relation to 'older' subjectivities and the 'forms of moral subjectivation and the practices of self that are meant to ensure it' (Foucault, 1990b: 29). Foucault used four analytic tools to interrogate the ethical domain: the ethical substance, the mode of subjection, the practices used to perform work on the self, and the desired mode of being. These elements constitute four 'folds' of subjectivation and provide useful tools for analysing the formation of 'older' subjectivities in relation to cosmetic surgery as a practice of self-care.

Ethical substance

The first element of subjectivation is the ethical substance, which constitutes the 'prime material of moral practice' (Foucault, 1990b: 26). The ethical substance is therefore formed by the part of the self that needs to be worked over to achieve moral conduct, described by Dean (1996: 222) as a 'materiality drenched in thought'. What Dean is suggesting is that the part of the self that is acted upon is material rendered intelligible and thus governable. In Western societies, the knowledge used to render objects and subjects intelligible tends to be produced through scientific disciplines and is thus linked to essentialist conceptions of the subject through games of truth and norms. Chapter 3 takes up analysis of the discourses that constitute the ageing of the older body as the 'ethical substance' in relation to cosmetic surgery practice.

Mode of subjection

The second element of subjectivation relates to the principles evoked in the work of the self upon the ethical substance. This is the mode of subjection, or 'the way in which the individual establishes his relation to the rule and recognises himself as obliged to put it into practice' (Foucault, 1990b: 27). As Dean (1996: 224) explains, the mode of subjectivation is concerned with 'the position we take or are given in relation to rules and norms, [and] with why we govern ourselves or others in a particular manner'. Deleuze (1986) describes the rules or norms contained by the mode of subjection as the 'snag' by which the folding of subjectivation occurs. In contemporary Western society these rules and norms tend to be produced by the human sciences and support a 'hermeneutics of the subject' which compels the ethical subject to form in relation to scientific knowledge and normative identities. This idea is put to work in Chapter 3 in order to examine the games of truth that constitute the subject in relation to 'older' and cosmetic surgery.

Practice of self

Practices of self are those used to perform 'ethical work' on the material substance and are the third element in Foucault's theorization of subjectivation. Practices of self support the mode of subjection and are undertaken to 'bring one's conduct into compliance with a given rule' and thus 'transform oneself into the ethical subject of one's behaviour' (Foucault, 1990b: 27).

Foucault (1994g: 225) also refers to these practices as 'technologies of self' which he elaborates as those:

> which permit individuals to effect by their own means, or with the help of others, a certain number of operations on their own bodies and souls, thoughts, conduct, and way of being, so as to transform themselves in order to attain a certain state of happiness, purity, wisdom, perfection, or immortality.

Foucault (1994g: 225) suggests that these 'technologies' are associated with a 'matrix of practical reason'. He writes, 'forms of rationality inscribe themselves in practices or systems of practices, and what role they play within them, because it's true that "practices" don't exist without a certain regimen of rationality' (Foucault, 1991b: 79). In the domain of ethics, true discourses are made to function as rational principles of action, or *logos* (Rabinow, 2003). Practices of self, therefore, bind the subject to a truth through the transformation of the individual into an ethical subject and can therefore be understood as a way of acting and thinking at once. Given this conceptualization, practices of self 'provide the intelligibility key for the correlative constitution of the subject and the object' (Florence, 1994: 463). This third element of subjectivation is critical to reconceptualizing cosmetic surgery as a practice of self. The methodological imperative suggested by this theorization is to interrogate cosmetic surgery in terms of the regimen of rationality inscribed in its practice in relation to 'older' people, which occurs in Chapter 4.

Telos

The fourth element of subjectivation in Foucault's theorization pertains to the mode of being or *telos* that the subject strives to attain through ethical conduct. As Foucault (1990b: 28) elaborates, moral action 'commits an individual, not only to other actions always in conformity with values and rules, but to a certain mode of being, a mode characteristic of the ethical subject'. The goal of ethical action is therefore 'not simply "self-awareness" but self-formation as an "ethical subject"' (Foucault, 1990b: 28). Foucault's analyses of the Greco-Roman texts illustrate how in stylizing the self as an ethical subject, life is given form through a stylistics of existence. This was encapsulated by the concept of *technē tou biou* - the arts of existence that enabled one to constitute a life of virtue. As Foucault (1990b: 28) explains, 'all moral action involves a relationship with the reality in which it is carried out, and a relationship with the self'. What this suggests is that practices of self and a mode of living are mutually implicated such that 'The practice of the self is identified and united with the art of living itself' (Foucault, 2005: 205). Deleuze (1986: 104) suggests that this constitutes the 'ultimate fold', the 'fold of the outside itself' which 'constitutes an "interiority of expectation" from which the subject, in different ways, hopes for immortality, eternity, salvation, freedom or death or detachment'. This final element of subjectivation is deployed in Chapter 5 to explore how 'older' is constituted in terms of a desirable mode of being linked to 'lifestyle'.

The significance of care of self for a new ethic of 'older'

Foucault's analysis of the relations established between the subject and truth were undertaken in an effort to demonstrate how, through inherent contingency according to conditions of possibility, things could be 'otherwise'. Methodologically, this strategy is informed by his conception of resistance whereby acts of resistance force modification to existing relations of power (Foucault, 1988b, Foucault, 1994f), that enable the promotion of new forms of subjectivity. Drawing on his reading of Foucault, Gabardi (2001:76) writes:

> The idea of an ethics of resistance that developed out of his analysis of the power/resistance relationship involved forging a "discipline of resistance" against a specific "disciplinary matrix" of domination. The fashioning of a resistant type of power through strategically chosen practices of self- transformation requires an ethos of disciplined freedom.

What Gabardi is suggesting is that acts of resistance entail critical engagement with practices of self. Foucault (2005: 252) writes, 'there is no first or final point of resistance to political power other than in the relationship one has to oneself'. From this statement it is apparent that Foucault intended the ethic of 'care of the self' to inform a general strategy of critical resistance.

Given that 'care of the self' entailed critical reflection, Rabinow (2003: 10) observes that it 'was also a form of critique, a critique of the self that entailed perpetual self examination'. Such a critique entails reflection upon how we are disciplined with respect to our identities and courses of action in order to test the limits of these forms of subjectivity and relations of power (Gabardi, 2001). The practice of critique thus provides 'a means of contesting the identities constructed by experts, abstract systems and dominant groups' (Dean, 1996: 214). Lloyd (1996: 250, emphasis in original) argues that 'self- fashioning, *when allied to critique*, can produce sites of contestation over the meanings and contours of identity, and over the ways in which certain practices are mobilized'. That sites of contestation over meaning can be generated by critique is in line with Foucault's conception of resistance and his proclamation that 'discourse is the power which is to be seized' (Foucault, 1981: 211). Moreover, Lloyd is suggesting that through critical engagement, the rationality associated with practices of self can be negotiated or influenced. This latitude of movement, or slippage of meaning, is a strategic means for transforming the present.

Read through Foucault's conceptualization of care of self as an ethical practice of critique, this book suggests that whilst cosmetic surgery may inscribe and reinscribe normative forms of subjectivity, its practice might also be understood in terms of transforming the self. As previously established, in contemporary somatic ethics 'care of self' is undertaken through practices used to fashion and care for the body. Practices of body modification such as cosmetic surgery can therefore be read as practices of self. According to Foucault's theorization of subjectivation, practices of self are engaged to constitute oneself as an ethical subject but are also a means for contesting identities and shaping new and modified subjectivities. For Foucault, the practice of critique is linked to the desire to resist modes of government. This is not a question of refusing all government but rather an imperative relating to 'how not to be governed like that, by that, in the name of those principles, with such and such an objective in mind and by means of such procedures, not like that, not for that, not by them' (Foucault, 1997a: 28). Critique however, does not necessarily take the form of a deduction that concludes what needs to be done. Foucault (1991b: 84) is precise in his statement that 'It should be an instrument for those who fight, those who resist and refuse what is....It doesn't have to lay down the law for the law. It isn't a stage in a programming. It's a challenge directed to what is'.

Foucault considered the practice of critique a virtue, linked to an ethos of what it means to be and how being might be experienced differently. This is what Foucault (1997b: 132) refers to as 'the critical ontology of ourselves'. The strategic insight offered by Foucault, that the limits of thought have an uncertain foundation in conditions of possibility, creates the potential that things might be 'otherwise' and thus critique 'does not mark out impassable boundaries or describe closed systems; it brings to light transformable singularities' (Foucault, 1994e: 201). The aim of a critical ontology of the self is to 'separate out from the contingency that has made us what we are, the possibility of no longer being, doing, or thinking what we are, do or think' (Foucault, 1997b: 125). The importance of this, as Foucault (1988c: 155) explains, is that 'as soon as one can no longer think things as one formerly thought them, transformation becomes both very urgent, very difficult, and quite possible'.

The possibility of transforming the self is enmeshed with processes that form the subject as an object for itself. The mode by which the self forms itself 'otherwise' is through ethical practices. As Butler (2001: 9) explains, 'there is no possibility of accepting or refusing a rule without a self who is stylized in response to the ethical demand upon it'. The transformation of the self thus occurs in relation to ethical precepts. In Foucault's conceptualization of ethics, the reflexive relation of self to self forms at a nexus between aesthetics, ethical principles and critique. Through the practice of critique it becomes possible to 'produce a subject who is not readily knowable under the established rubric of truth' (Butler, 2001: 12). As Butler (2001: 20) elaborates:

> if that self-forming is done in disobedience to the principles by which one is formed, then virtue becomes the practice by which the self forms in desubjugation, which is to say that it risks its deformation as a subject occupying that ontologically insecure position which poses the question anew: who will be a subject here, and what will count as a life, a moment

> of ethical questioning which requires that we break the habits of judgement in favour of a riskier practice that seeks to yield artistry from constraint.

According to Butler, in this 'moment of ethical questioning' there is a 'contingent, even free, moment' where the form of ethical relation to self is open to artistic licence (Butler and Connolly, 2000: 17). As Foucault (1994b: 284) proclaims, 'Freedom is the ontological condition of ethics. But ethics is the considered form that freedom takes when informed by reflection'. Ethics is thus a response to the problem of how freedom is practiced and the self is given form. Through aesthetic self-stylization the subject may exceed the limitations of 'truth', or as Foucault (1997a: 32) writes, 'Critique would essentially ensure the desubjugation of the subject in the context of what we could call, in a word, the politics of truth'. Foucault's work on ancient ethics thus provides the 'concepts with which to analyse an ethics of freedom' (Rabinow, 2003: 45). Adopting this position draws analytic attention to the ways in which agency, freedom and resistance are performed through the body using cosmetic surgery to stylize appearance, mode of being and experience of life in ways that challenge the normative and taken-for-granted rendering of 'older'.

Empirical data and its analysis

The empirical texts used in the analyses in this book were generated in a research project that was granted ethical approval by the University of South Australia and data were collected in Adelaide, Sydney and Brisbane. Qualitative research methods were used in the study to generate media articles on older people and cosmetic surgery and interview data with people who had undergone cosmetic surgery whilst aged 65–75 years and cosmetic surgeons and practitioners. These textual data serve as sites for purposively sampling the discourses that shape interpretations of 'older' in relation to cosmetic surgery. 'Popular' print media was selected in the study to enable analysis of contemporary representations of cosmetic surgery engaged in by 'older people' including newspaper, magazine and online articles in broad public circulation nationally and internationally. Online databases and the internet were searched using keywords to locate information rich articles. The retrieved articles span the years 1992–2008 (see Table 2.1).

Two participant groups were recruited for the study. Participants who had undergone cosmetic surgery ranged from 66 years to 75 years (n = 11). The majority (n = 8) were female which reflects the gender imbalance amongst cosmetic surgery consumers. A diverse range of cosmetic procedures including surgical and medical procedures were represented in the sample with some participants having undergone multiple procedures (see Table 2.2).

In the practitioner group (n = 10) there were an even number of males and females (see Table 2.3). Four participants worked in the field of plastic

Table 2.1 Chronology of media texts (1992–2008)

Author & date published	*Heading & source*
Jane Hass (1992) 27th December	Approach cosmetic surgery with your eyes wide open *The Dallas Morning News* (USA)
Robert Stock (1996) 25th July	Senior class: face-lift surgery gains adherents *The New York Times* (New York, USA)
Patsy Crawford (1999) 30th May	Should be the year of facelift *Sunday Tasmanian* (Tasmania, Australia)
Garry Linnell (1999) 16th November	You Beauty *Bulletin within Newsweek* (Australia)
Valerie Grove (2000) 26th February	'Under the knife, I find the real me' *The Times* (London, UK)
No Author (2000) 27th October	Young in heart, mind, body – and face *Toronto Star* (Canada)
Carol Potera (2000) 18th December	Turning back time: new face, new outlook Article on *MedicineNet.com* (USA)
Denise Ryan (2001) 17th December	Adding years gracefully – Mind & body – ageing *The Age* (Melbourne, Australia)
Lisette Hilton (2002) 1st June	Older Americans have special cosmetic surgery needs *Cosmetic Surgery Times Special Reports* (USA)
No Author (2002) 24th July	More people 65 and older getting cosmetic surgery *The Canadian Press* (Canada)
Colleen Long (2002) 1st August	Forever young *CBS News online* (USA)
Nicki Daniels (2002) 12th November	So what's wrong with wrinkles? – Lifetime *The Times* (London, UK)
Megan Norris (2003) 17th February	60 years of plastic surgery: But her love is blind *Women's Day* (Australia)
Julie Robotham (2004) 29th March	Boomers keep raising eyebrows *The Sydney Morning Herald* (Sydney, Australia)
Janet Kornblum (2004) 25th May	'I wanted to look how I feel' *USA Today* (USA)
Helen Fields (2004) 18th October	Cosmetic surgery: time for grandma to get a face lift? *US News and World Report* (USA)
Lee Tulloch (2004) November	Facing the Future *Australian Women's Weekly* (Australia)
The British Association of Aesthetic Plastic Surgeons (2005) 21st March	Plastic surgery: it's not teens, it's their grandparents! *The British Association of Aesthetic Plastic Surgeons* (UK)
No Author (2005) 23rd March	Grandparents turn to cosmetic ops *BBC News Online* (UK)

Table 2.1 (continued)

Author & date published	*Heading & source*
No Author (2005) 28th March	Seniors like to 'nip and tuck' *Medical Research News* (UK)
Maxine Frith (2005) 28th March	Holding back the years: how the older generation fell for cosmetic *The Independent* (London, UK)
No Author (2005) 27th April	New bodies for old souls *Panipatonline* (UK)
No Author (2005) 9th May	Cosmetic surgery rise for over 50s *The Independent* (London, UK)
No Author (2005) 11th June	Older generation looking younger *DukeMedNews online* (USA)
Allen-Mills (2005) 24th July	Grandads join the facelift set *The Sunday Times* (London, UK)
John Jesitus (2006) March	Age before beauty? What age is too young or old? *Cosmetic Surgery Times* (USA)
Jenny Brown (2006) 24th April	'I'm 85 and still love plastic surgery' *Women's Day* (Australia)
Alan Hamilton (2006) 29th May	Not-so-wrinklies line up for facelifts *The Times* (London, UK)
Julie Wheldon (2006) 29th May	Silver surgery surge *Daily Mail* (UK)
No Author (2006) 31st May	Cosmetic surgery for the elderly *Alphamaleblog* (unknown origin)
No Author (2006) 29th November	Cosmetic surgery helps to make sixties new middle age *MedicalSearch online* (Australia)
Media Monitors (2007) 2nd February	5AA radio transcript of interview by Amanda Blair with Dr Daniel Fleming (Australia)
American Society of Plastic Surgeons (2007) 22nd March	Cosmetic plastic surgery for baby boomers shifts to lifts *ASPS press release* (USA)
Rosemary Gallagher (2007) 24th February	Older people looking at a surgically enhanced retirement *The Scotsman* (UK)
Virginia Ironside (2007) 3rd May	Sexy to be wrinkly? So why have you had all that work done, Jane? *Daily Mail* (UK)
Emma Pinch (2008) 17th January	The rise of silver surgery *Liverpool Daily Post* (UK)

Table 2.2 Participant profiles: 'older' people who have undergone cosmetic surgery

Pseudonym	*Profile*
Angela	Angela is aged 67 and is retired but does volunteer work at a hospital. She shares her home with a boarder and is a keen gardener. At the time of the interview she was waiting for a shoulder operation and had been experiencing some health difficulties generally. She had been recommended abdominoplasty but decided to have liposuction given the lower risks and less invasive processes involved. The decision to have the procedure was informed by both cosmetic and medical reasons to reduce her weight and was self-financed.
Charlotte	Charlotte is 69 years of age and lives with her retired partner. She works in the travel industry and is also with a casting agency but their main income is derived from property investments. She has undergone cosmetic surgery a number of times during her life including breast augmentation when she was younger (the augmentation was subsequently reversed), a facelift when she was in her forties, skin resurfacing, liposuction and most recently (three months prior to the interview) she had work done around her chin to reduce her jowls. She thinks that her drive to look her best comes from feelings of insecurity that stem from her childhood experiences of being raised by different family members at various times.
Chloe	Chloe is 70 years of age and lives with her partner of 44 years with whom she has three children. She works full time in her own business and lives in an up market area. She describes her lifestyle as busy and through her work travels a great deal. Chloe had liposculture of her abdomen and considered this as being different to having cosmetic surgery of the face which she saw as being related to identity. Given that she is busy and active she does not consider herself old at 70 but thinks that younger people would see her that way.
Chris	Chris is aged 70 and is semi-retired but about to become fully retired. He feels ambivalent about this change because he relates his identity to his career and does not want to become a 'pensioner'. He considers himself to be a young 70 year old and does not relate to the activities he considers older people like to engage in such as playing cards or bowling. He had cosmetic surgery to lift the corners of either side of his mouth and states that if he had the money he would get his eyelids and stomach done.
Emily	Emily is 68 and lives alone. She is not particularly interested in activities related to her appearance. However she underwent eye surgery, both her eyelid and underneath her eyes, because her drooping eyelids were reminding her of her mother and she wanted to improve her appearance.
Heather	Heather is aged 69 and lives alone in a unit. She works for an agency organizing shift workers. She has a chronic illness that she manages and considers herself fit from playing sport. Heather considers herself a spiritual person and sees age as just a number. She suggests that keeping the mind and body active is what is important. She sees a cosmetic physician to have laser treatment of her face and has chemical peels regularly.

Table 2.2 (continued)

Pseudonym	*Profile*
Isabella	Isabella is aged 75, lives alone and is retired and receiving a pension. She has a large extended family and considers herself very active. Over quite a long period of time beginning with neck surgery, she had face peels, eyelid surgery and liposuction. She had to work hard to save up the money for the procedures but considers it worth the expense to feel comfortable with herself.
James	James is aged 72 years old and has been retired for 11 years. He lives with his partner of 25 years in a retirement village. He told me that since he has very good health and is an active person, with golf and bushwalking as hobbies, he does not consider himself to be old although sometimes he realizes he is getting older. James had two cosmetic procedures: surgery for gynecomastia but this left his chest 'creased' and so he had another procedure to improve the appearance of his chest.
Mandy	Mandy is 66 years of age and a widow of six years. She lives alone on a large property in a big house which she has been renovating (a pool was being installed at the time of the interview) and she does a lot of travel. Over a 12 month period she had a tummy tuck, breast reduction, liposuction of her thighs and mini facelift. She was originally motivated to have the breast reduction due to health complications but also wanted to wear and look good in stylish clothes.
Sophie	Sophie is aged 70 and is a widow of 12 years. She has many complex health difficulties and these are preventing her from having any further cosmetic surgery. Sophie had a facelift when she was 45 and more recently has undergone facial rejuvenation procedures including laser treatment, chemical peels and fat transfer for her face and neck.
Tom	Tom is aged 70 and lives with his second wife. He is semi-retired in that he undertakes paid work part time but he has also remained involved in the industry in which his career was based. He contributes to his community through involvement in functions and hosts high profile guests to Australia. He has undergone body contouring procedures for his abdomen, jaw line and nose and most recently a thread lift. Tom's appearance is important to him in the context of his active social and public life and in terms of wanting to look good.

Table 2.3 Participant profiles: cosmetic surgery practitioners

Pseudonym	*Profile*
Dr Brown	Dr Brown is a cosmetic physician with a general practice background that led to an interest in surgery. He works in the area of cosmetic medicine and performs a number of procedures but has a specialist area of expertise. He finds cosmetic work rewarding because it helps people to feel better and is passionate about the advancement of the field. He feels that older people engage in cosmetic surgery to enhance their looks so that they feel confident in social relations.
Dr Cooper	Dr Cooper is a plastic surgeon who works part time in public hospital practice and part time in private practice. He performs both plastic and cosmetic procedures and considers aesthetic surgery to be a sub- specialty of plastic surgery. Dr Cooper considers cosmetic surgery to produce small increases in quality of life in a society that is generally well-off. He regards older people undergoing cosmetic surgery as doing something for themselves and trying to realign their appearance with how they feel.
Ms Harris	Ms Harris is a personal assistant to a plastic surgeon whose practice is comprised of approximately 60% cosmetic work encompassing a broad range of procedures. Her role is to provide patients with quotes and information and essentially operate as the conduit between patients and the surgeon unless a direct consultation is required. She sees cosmetic surgery as a matter of individual ethics but personally feels it is an unnecessary risk especially for older people whose advanced ageing might also compromise the success of the procedure.
Ms Robinson	Ms Robinson owns/operates a beauty salon in the same building as a high status hairdressing salon that has the relaxed contemporary feel of a day spa. The salon offers beauty treatments and therapies and some cosmetic medicine including injection procedures. Ms Robinson believes that cosmetic surgery is driven by insecurities we have about ourselves but directed at the body and that failed relationships are a large impetus for women undergoing cosmetic surgery. She was sceptical about whether older people would be undergoing cosmetic surgery because she felt that by ages 65–75 people have accepted themselves for who they are and are no longer looking for new relationships.
Dr Smith	Dr Smith is a cosmetic physician with a general practice background. She currently operates a private practice that focuses on cosmetic medicine and minor surgical procedures. Her premises are located in a wealthy suburb close to the central business district and combine elements of design from a small general practice environment (particularly her consulting room layout) with the beauty industry (particularly the attention paid to the aesthetics of the reception and waiting room). The majority of Dr Smith's patients are 40–60 years of age but she also has patients who are older than that. She views cosmetic surgery amongst older people as indicative of social changes and also ageism.

Table 2.3 continued

Pseudonym	*Profile*
Ms Taylor	Ms Taylor is the practice manager at a plastic surgery practice. The practice includes multiple surgeons and covers a range of medical and surgical cosmetic procedures and plastic surgery procedures. Ms Taylor felt that cosmetic surgery is an individual consumer choice and largely frivolous, which differentiates it from medically indicated plastic surgery. She attributed the increasing numbers of older people undergoing cosmetic surgery to increasing longevity and social and cultural emphases on looking good, fitness and health.
Ms Martin	Ms Martin is a personal assistant to a plastic surgeon whose practice focuses on cosmetic procedures. As part of her role she meets with patients to draw up quotes, provide post-operative information and organize medical garments. Ms Martin does not promote cosmetic surgery because she feels people do not need it and should be happy with themselves. However, she also believes in individual consumer choice and links the increasing numbers of older people having cosmetic procedures to affluence and desire to 'do something for myself'.
Dr Watts	Dr Watts is a cosmetic surgeon with a background in surgical and plastic surgery training. His area of specialty is breast augmentation but he practices a range of cosmetic procedures. The consultation rooms in which he works have a contemporary relaxed feel incorporating bold colours, artwork and plants. Dr Watts regards cosmetic surgery as a specialty area undertaken by doctors but one that is shaped by market forces. He believes that older people are seeking cosmetic surgery because they want to look as good as they feel.
Dr Williams	Dr Williams is a cosmetic surgeon with a general surgery background in the public hospital system. He specializes in body contouring procedures including liposuction, liposculpture and breast surgeries. Dr Williams believes that cosmetic surgery is important for promoting self esteem but does not see this as being so important for older patients. From his experience he believes that older patients are particularly interested in minimally invasive procedures that result in a more youthful look, being more comfortable and having clothes fit better.
Dr Wilson	Dr Wilson is a cosmetic surgeon with a background in cardiothoracic surgery whose current cosmetic practice focuses on facial procedures. Dr Wilson is passionate about the creative and artistic aspects of the craft of aesthetic surgery. He believes that older consumers of cosmetic surgery are trying to enhance their appearance and look closer to an appearance that they have lost over time.

surgery, five were cosmetic surgeons or physicians and one was a beauty therapist who owns and operates a business offering a range of cosmetic medical procedures.

A semi-structured approach was taken to conducting the interviews in this study (Patton, 2002). This meant that the interview guide provided the topics, and example questions, but these were used flexibly to explore, probe, word questions spontaneously, and move amongst topics with the flow of the interview as it unfolded. The interview schedule was designed to elicit discourses that constitute 'older' subjectivities and cosmetic surgery practice and those that shape interpretations of older people who undergo cosmetic surgery.

The theoretical analysis undertaken in this book constitutes a meditation on how the ontology of 'older' and the practice of cosmetic surgery are discursively constructed and the contemporary contexts that shape these discourses. This labour of meditation entails practices of thinking as a method of analysis (Deacon, 2000). Through a focus on discourse, the object of this thinking, however, is not a referent but thought itself. The analytic chapters presented in this book thus take up 'interpretations of interpretations' (Foucault, 1994c: 276). As Foucault (1994c: 275) suggests:

> if interpretation can never be completed, this is quite simply because there is nothing to interpret, for after all everything is already interpretation, each sign is in itself not the thing that offers itself to interpretation but an interpretation of other signs.

Taking thought as the object for critical work and reflecting on it as a problem demands an 'unrelenting scepticism' of 'truth' on the basis of discourse (Hook, 2001: 524). Foucault termed this critical work problematization; which refers to both that which was the focus of his analysis as well as his analytic approach. The methodological imperative suggested here is to 'problematize' that which has become normative and taken-for-granted by revealing the historical conditions – the conditions of possibility – required to establish something as universal, necessary and self-evident, in short, to problematize that which is established as 'truth'.

Summary

Drawing on Foucault's thought in relation to ethics, the political ambition of this book entails a 'suspension of the regimen of truth that governs the elaboration and totalization of identities' (Butler & Connolly, 2000: 9). The aesthetic and ethical ambition realised in such a task is to open up 'older' and the practice of cosmetic surgery by 'older' people to alternative interpretation. Rather than consider the ontology of 'older' from the angle of knowledge, it is to be considered 'instead from the angle of practice, of the exercise of self on self...in a realm that is no longer one of truth' (Foucault, 2005: 317) but of ethics. A dynamic nexus between theory and empirical data provides the approach and framework for the chapters to follow. This approach enables the problematization of normative discourses of 'ageing', 'anti-ageing' and 'denial of ageing' and provides the conceptual resources for understanding *becoming* 'older' through critical and reflexive self-stylization in relation to cosmetic surgery.

Notes

1 In *The Order of Things* Foucault makes the infamous claim that 'man is an invention of recent date. And one perhaps nearing its end' (p.387).
2 'Subjectivation' sometimes translated as 'subjectification' is the term Foucault uses to refer to the processes through which a subject is constituted.
3 In *What is Enlightenment*, Foucault (1997c: 118) draws on Baudelaire to suggest '*dandysme*' is a form of aesthetic practice whereby the dandy 'makes of his body, his behaviour, his feelings and passions, his very existence, a work of art'.

References

Barry, A., Osborne, T. & Rose, N. 1996. *Foucault and Political Reason: Liberalism, Neo-Liberalism, and Rationalities of Government*. Chicago: University of Chicago Press.

Baudrillard, J. 1998. *The Consumer Society: Myths & Structures.* London: Sage Publications.

Bauman, Z. 2007. *Consuming Life*. Cambridge: Polity Press.

Bauman, Z. 2008. *The Art of Life*. Cambridge: Polity Press.

Besley, T. A. C. & Peters, M. A. 2007. *Subjectivity and Truth: Foucault, Education and the Culture of the Self.* New York: Peter Lang Publishing.

Binkley, S. 2007. Governmentality and Lifestyle Studies. *Sociology Compass*, 1, 111–126.

Butler, J. 1997. *The Psychic Life of Power: Theories in Subjection*. Stanford: Stanford University Press.

Butler, J. 2001. *What is Critique? An Essay on Foucault's Virtue* [Online]. Available: http://www.law.berkeley.edu/centers/kadish/what%20is%20critique%20J%20Butler.pdf [Accessed 30 August 2006].

Butler, J. & Connolly, W. 2000. Politics, Power and Ethics: A Discussion between Judith Butler and William Connolly. *Theory & Event*, 4, 28.

Davidson, A. I. 2005. Introduction. In: Gros, F. (ed.) *The Hermeneutics Of The Subject: Lectures at the College De France 1981–1982*. New York: Picador.

Deacon, R. 2000. Theory as Practice: Foucault's Concept of Problematization. *Telos*, 118, 127–142.

Dean, M. 1996. Foucault, Government and the Enfolding of Authority. In: Barry, A., Osborne, T. & Rose, N. (eds) *Foucault and Political Reason: Liberalism, Neo-liberalism and Rationalities of Government*. Chicago: The University of Chicago Press.

Deleuze, G. 1986. *Foucault*. Minneapolis: University of Minnesota Press.

Dreyfus, H. L. & Rabinow, P. 1982. *Michel Foucault: Beyond Structuralism and Hermeneutics.* Chicago: The University of Chicago Press.

Featherstone, M. 2007. *Consumer Culture and Postmodernism.* London: Sage Publications.

Fillion, R. 2005. Freedom, Truth, and Possibility in Foucault's Ethics. *Foucault Studies*, 3, 50–64.

Florence, M. 1994. Foucault. In: Faubion, J. D. (ed.) *Michel Foucault: Aesthetics, Method and Epistemology*. New York: The New Press.

Foucault, M. 1961. *Madness and Civilization: A History of Insanity in the Age of Reason*. Cambridge: Routledge.

Foucault, M. 1972. *The Archaeology of Knowledge and the Discourse on Language*. New York: Pantheon Books.

Foucault, M. 1976. *The Will to Knowledge: The History of Sexuality Volume 1*. London: Penguin Books.

Foucault, M. 1981. The Order of Discourse. In: Young, R. (ed.) *Untying The Text: A Post-Structuralist Reader*. Boston: Routledge & Kegan Paul.

Foucault, M. 1984. Nietzsche, Genealogy, History. In: Rabinow, P. (ed.) *The Foucault Reader: An Introduction to Foucault's Thought*. New York: Random House.

Foucault, M. 1988a. An Aesthetics of Existence. In: Kritzman, L. D. (ed.) *Michel Foucault: Politics, Philosophy, Culture: Interviews and other Writings 1977–1984*. New York: Routledge.

Foucault, M. 1988b. Power and Sex. In: Kritzman, L. D. (ed.) *Michel Foucault. Politics, Philosophy, Culture: Interviews and other Writings 1977–184*. New York: Routledge.

Foucault, M. 1988c. Practicing Criticism. In: Kritzman, L. D. (ed.) *Michel Foucault. Politics, Philosophy, Culture: Interviews and other Writings 1977–1984*. New York: Routledge.

Foucault, M. 1989. *The Order of Things*. New York: Routledge.

Foucault, M. 1990a. *The Care of the Self: The History of Sexuality Volume 3*. London: Penguin Books.

Foucault, M. 1990b. *The Use of Pleasure: The History of Sexuality Volume 2*. USA: Vintage Books.

Foucault, M. 1991a. *Discipline and Punish: The Birth of the Prison*. Harmondsworth: Penguin.

Foucault, M. 1991b. Questions of Method. In: Burchell, G., Gordon, C. & Miller, P. (eds) *The Foucault Effect: Studies in Governmentality*. Hertfordshire: Harvester Wheatsheaf.

Foucault, M. 1994a. The Ethic of Care for the Self as a Practice of Freedom. In: Bernauer, J. & Rasmussen, D. (eds) *The Final Foucault*. Cambridge: The MIT Press.

Foucault, M. 1994b. The Ethics of the Concern with the Self as a Practice of Freedom. In: Rabinow, P. (ed.) *Michel Foucault: Ethics, Subjectivity and Truth*. New York: The New Press.

Foucault, M. 1994c. Nietzsche, Freud, Marx. In: Fabion, J. D. (ed.) *Michel Foucault: Aesthetics, Method and Epistemology*. New York: The New York Press.

Foucault, M. 1994d. On the Genealogy of Ethics: An Overview of a Work in Progress. In: Rabinow, P. (ed.) *Michel Foucault: Ethics, Subjectivity and Truth*. New York: The New York Press.

Foucault, M. 1994e. *Preface to the History of Sexuality, Volume Two*. In: Rabinow, P. (ed.) *Michel Foucault: Ethics, Subjectiviity and Truth*. New York: The New Press.

Foucault, M. 1994f. Sex, Power and the Politics of Identity. In: Rabinow, P. (ed.) *Michel Foucault: Ethics, Subjectivity and Truth*. New York: The New Press.

Foucault, M. 1994g. Subjectivity and Truth. In: Rabinow, P. (ed.) *Michel Foucault: Ethics, Subjectivity and Truth*. New York: The New Press.

Foucault, M. 1997a. What is Critique? In: Lotringer, S. & Hochroth, L. (eds) *The Politics of Truth*. USA: The MIT Press.

Foucault, M. 1997b. What is Enlightenment? In: Lotringer, S. & Hochroth, L. (eds) *The Politics of Truth*. USA: Semiotext(e).

Foucault, M. 2005. *The Hermeneutics of the Subject: Lectures at the College De France 1981–1982*. New York: Picador.

Gabardi, W. 2001. *Negotiating Postmodernism*. Minneapolis: University of Minnesota Press.

Gros, F. 2005. Course Context. In: Gros, F. (ed.) *The Hermeneutics of the Subject: Lectures at the College de France 1981–1982*. New York: Palgrave Macmillian.

Hamann, T. H. 2009. Neoliberalism, Governmentality, and Ethics. *Foucault Studies*, 6, 37–59.

Hook, D. 2001. Discourse, Knowledge, Materiality, History: Foucault and Discourse Analysis. *Theory & Psychology*, 11, 521–547.

Lloyd, M. 1996. A Feminist Mapping of Foucauldian Politics. In: Hekman, S. J. (ed.) *Feminist Interpretations of Michel Foucault*. Pennsylvania: The Pennsylvania State University Press.

N.A. 2005. *New Bodies for Old Souls* [Online]. PanipatOnline.com. Available: www.panipatonline.com/article_read.asp?id=1896 [Accessed 13 March 2008].

Paras, E. 2006. *Foucault 2.0: Beyond Power and Knowledge*. New York: Other Press.

Patton, M. Q. 2002. *Qualitative Research & Evaluation Methods*. California: Sage Publications.

Probyn, E. 1993. *Sexing the Self: Gendered Positions in Cultural Studies*. London: Routledge.

Rabinow, P. 1994. The History of Systems of Thought. In: Rabinow, P. (ed.) *Michel Foucault: Ethics, Subjectivity and Truth*. New York: The New Press.

Rabinow, P. 2003. *Anthropos Today: Reflections on Modern Equipment*. New Jersey: Princeton University Press.

Rose, N. 2001. The Politics of Life Itself. *Theory, Culture & Society*, 18, *1–30*.

Rose, N. 2007. *The Politics of Life Itself: Biomedicine, Power, and Subjectivity in the Twenty-First Century*. New Jersey: Princeton University Press.

Rose, N. n.d. *Power in Therapy: Techne and Ethos* [Online]. Academy for the Study of the Psychoanalytic Arts. Available: http://www.academyanalyticarts.org/rose2.htm [Accessed 8 December 2009].

Ryan, D. 2001. Adding Years Gracefully. *The Age*.

Stock, R. W. 1996. Senior Class: Face-Lift Surgery Gains Adherents. *The New York Times*, 25 July.

Twigg, J. 2004. The Body, Gender, and Age: Feminist Insights in Social Gerontology. *Journal of Aging Studies*, 18, 59–73.

3 The fractured 'older' subject at the limits of 'ageing'

Introduction

The way in which the 'older' subject is 'put into discourse' (Foucault, 1976) in relation to cosmetic surgery is shaped by a normative system of inscription. This system comprises prevailing 'regimens of truth' (Foucault, 1990) that inscribe and problematize the 'older' subject in relation to an ethics of the self connected to 'ageing'. This chapter establishes that these dominant regimens of truth are an outworking of a Cartesian ethics that cleaves the subject into the rational transcendental mind and the natural material body (Grosz, 1994). The problem of this ethics in relation to 'ageing', is one in which the subjective experience of 'older' is fractured by dissonance between the 'ageing' body and the 'ageless' transcendental self. The chapter begins by drawing on themes, amplified through excerpts of data, to elaborate the ways in which the dissonance between body and self is articulated in the textual data and the extant literature on 'ageing'. To analyse how the self and body are rendered intelligible in ways that generate this dissonance, Foucault's theorization of the mode of subjection and ethical substance (see Chapter 2) is drawn upon in relation to an ethics of the self. The mode of subjection in cosmetic surgery discourse is explored in terms of the hermeneutics of the subject which installs the interiority of the subject and defines its relation to 'truth'. The focus is then directed to the 'body' to explore how the 'older' ageing body is objectified and rendered problematic through discourses of ageing. It is these discourses of ageing that constitute the normative body as 'youthful' and problematizes the 'older' body as the ethical substance to be worked over by the practice of cosmetic surgery. This normative and essentialist system of inscription thus remains anchored in the 'old discourses and dividing practices' (Gilleard and Higgs, 2013) of ageing that restrict possibilities for the embodiment of *becoming* 'older'.

Dissonance in ageing: the body and the subject in games of truth

A problematization of the congruence between the interiority of the 'self' and the physical body underpins accounts of cosmetic surgery by older people.

This problematization is articulated in terms of a dissonance between the 'ageing' of the body and a perceived sense of self that fractures the subjective experience of 'older' (see also Morton, 2015). Older people who have undergone cosmetic surgery, cosmetic surgery practitioners and media texts articulate this dissonance in terms of various intersections between chronological age, appearance of the body and sense of self.

For Charlotte, aged 69 years, the dissonance between her chronological age and appearance was the reason for her decision to undergo cosmetic surgery to tighten the area of her jowls because she 'felt she was looking older than my years'. This form of dissonance was referred to as 'premature ageing' and having 'aged beyond your years' by Dr Wilson and Dr Cooper. Such judgements concerning 'premature' ageing are based in normative thought concerning how bodies *should* appear at particular ages. In this way, norms render bodies intelligible in relation to age. However, in the 'games of truth' (Foucault, 1997) in which these norms operate, the chronological age of the subject anchors the normative appearance of the ageing body. That this game of truth is sustained and continually played out when the limits of its intelligibility are frequently rendered visible, when confronted with people who, without any surgical intervention to appearance, look 'older' or 'younger' than their 'actual' age, is testament to the power of norms.

Ms Taylor problematizes the normative fixing of an ageing appearance in her statement that 'some seventy year olds look like they're a hundred and you see others who look like they're fifty'. The following excerpt from a media article (The Canadian Press, 2002) specifically disconnects chronological age from appearance and sense of self in relation to cosmetic surgery practice. The article features Hazel York, an 81 year old living in California who underwent a facelift, and cites her surgeon as stating:

> Hazel's a perfect example that chronological age doesn't have to relate to how you feel about yourself. Just because you're 80 doesn't mean you have to look and feel like it.

What this statement does, is problematize chronological age in terms of determining how the body should appear or how the self should be experienced in relation to age. That this statement emerges in relation to cosmetic surgery practice connects the practice of body modification to a transformation of the norms connected to chronological age in relation to the embodied subject. This transformation is not limited to a surface plane from which the age of the body is 'read' but reveals a deeper problematization of the 'game of truth' through which the ageing subject is constituted, in which chronological age no longer holds the power of 'truth'.

Instability in normative judgements concerning ageing and appearance are an outworking of a modification to the ethics of ageing enabled by body modification practices such as cosmetic surgery. In the data generated for this book, the general form of problematization of the relation between self and body was not connected to chronological age but emerged as dissonance between outer appearance and inner feeling. As one media text (Daniels, 2002) put it, 'It is not that they look older than they are, but they look older than they feel'. As the following excerpts illustrate, self-perceptions of being young, fit and feeling good were presented as being in tension with an aged appearance as well as chronological age:

> Because their faces change. And what they see changes and they don't like it. I mean a lot of people say you know, 'I'm fifty' or whatever 'and I don't feel it at all. I am still active and fit and go to the gym and you know stand on my head and everything' and they look in the mirror. 'Don't like what I see'.
>
> (Dr Smith)

> What I find is that generally people feel quite energetic, they feel good. They might feel like they did when they were 20 or 30 but they look like they are 60. So there is a mismatch between how they look and feel. They look in the mirror and they see somebody who they don't feel like and so they may seek some redress to that.
>
> (Dr Watts)

This interpretation of dissonance concerns an inner feeling versus an outer appearance in relation to ageing. What excerpts such as these suggest is that whilst an inner experience of self remains constant and relatively 'youthful', bodily changes 'age' appearance creating the dissension between how the individual looks and feels. What remains unstated and thus taken for granted in these interpretations is why feeling energetic and good is necessarily incommensurate with the appearance of a 50 or 60 year old.

Another form of dissonance that emerged in the data is that between an inner feeling and outer expression of feeling as read by others. This form of dissonance is illustrated by a media extract in which a 67 year old female is reported as stating:

> What is annoying is that your mouth turns down and you get dewlaps. You may feel cheerful, but you look disagreeable and make people feel nervous. They interpret disapproval when it's not intended. So you just want to look more like you feel.
>
> (Grove, 2000)

What this excerpt suggests is that the physical body performs an expression that does not reflect inner feeling and thus misrepresents the self to others. This is an experience that Chris could relate to given his statement that 'every now and then my partner says to me you are looking a bit sour and I am not, but my facial structure is doing an old man's trick of sagging down'. In this statement, Chris specifically relates the source of the dissonance to an 'old man's' facial structure. In another interview, Dr Wilson attributes expression to corporeal ageing saying that 'the ageing process actually pushes the face down...eyebrows droop which creates a tired look or an angry look'. Ms Taylor offered the opinion in her interview that the reason older people have cosmetic surgery is because 'most of them just want to look not old and tired because they get people telling them they look tired all the time or sick – things like that'. The dissonance between outer expression and inner feeling illustrated by these examples is attributed to the ageing 'older' body. For Chris, cosmetic surgery is a practice that enabled him to address the tension between inner feeling and outer expression as he states 'I am not looking to look like an 18 year old, I want to look like a 65 year old, but so my face reflects my inside'.

For Chris, Chloe, Heather and Emily their sense of an 'inside' self was at odds with their chronological age or 'outside' body. Chris states that he is 'a younger person inside' and Heather tells me that 'you have got to remember, that even though I am 69 – I am talking about me now – in here I am still 16. I still think like I used to think'. Statements such as these create a division between the 'inside' and the 'outside' and indicate a tension between the perception of the self and the body in relation to ageing. This occurs because the 'inner' self is considered youthful and unchanging whilst the 'outer' body is seen to change with ageing. Chloe describes it thus, 'I don't think you move into old mentally, your body does but your mind doesn't. Most minds stay young.' Emily, aged 68, projects this formulation forward stating that 'I could be 80 and I'd still think the same way. I mean it's only old outside its not old in my head'. In these statements the body is the locus for 'ageing' through physical change whilst the self is fixed and relatively 'youthful'. Cosmetic surgery undertaken by 'older' people is therefore constituted as a practice – 'to make the stranger staring back at them in the mirror better reflect the youngster inside' (Pinch, 2008). Here the interior self is constituted as the 'truth' that is betrayed by the ageing body and restored by cosmetic surgery. As one 67 year old is reported to have said following facelift surgery, 'I have myself back again' (Stock, 1996).

In academic scholarship it has long been recognized that 'older' people draw a distinction between their ageing body, particularly in terms of appearance, and their internal sense of an 'ageless self' (Kaufman, 1986). Conceptualized as the 'mask of aging' (Featherstone and Hepworth, 1991: 379), this experience is interpreted as one in which the 'mask' of the ageing body 'conceals the essential identity of the person beneath'. Through the 'mask of aging', the ageing 'older' body is interpreted as creating a dissonance between 'self on the inside' and 'self presented to others'. That many consumers of cosmetic surgery constitute their experience through a 'mask of ageing' discourse was also evident in the literature (Askegaard, Gertsen and Langer, 2002; Blum, 2003; Gimlin, 2000). The 'mask of ageing' is therefore an academic discourse that reinscribes the fracture of the subject in relation to ageing and requires further critical examination.

Cartesian dualism and an essentialist ethic of ageing

The analysis presented here is evidence of an essentialist 'ethics of ageing' that governs how the 'older' subject forms in relation to discourses of ageing. This ethic is underpinned by the logos of Cartesian dualism which enacts a separation between the body and the self. Beginning with René Descartes, the logics of Cartesian dualism divided the subject of Western epistemology into the rational non-material mind, positioned outside the natural order, and the material body which given its 'naturalness' became the object of study in the human sciences (Grosz, 1994). The logics of Western scientific epistemology are connected to modernity and produce 'metanarratives that claim to capture universal processes underlying essential differences' (Powell and Longino, 2002: 222). This essentialist mode of ethics, associated with the scientific organization of knowledge, anchors a relationship between the subject and truth in which 'one of the main moral obligations for any subject is to know oneself, to tell the truth about oneself, and to constitute oneself as an object of knowledge both for other people and for oneself' (Foucault, 1997: 177). The human sciences thus impose a truth obligation upon the subject to be constituted as an object of scientific knowledge in relation to what has been established as 'normal' and 'natural'.

As Twigg (2004: 64) observes, the mask of ageing is an outworking of Cartesian dualism 'in which the self is seen as radically separate from the body, something that rises above it and remains disassociated from the body's corporeality'. Tulle-Winton (2000: 76) argues that the 'mask of ageing' is a strategy used by 'older' people to preserve their sense of self:

> The Cartesian dualism here was exploited and primacy given to the mind, confirmed as the seat of the self. The bodily signs of old age were reinterpreted as the mask which conveyed senescence and obsolescence and beneath which the true person, the real self, lay untouched, unchanged, unadulterated and timeless.

Öberg (2003: 106) suggests, that the 'mask of ageing' therefore 'offers a strategy for maintaining a positive and youthful self-concept'. The ethics of ageing enabled by Cartesian dualism thus enables the corporeality of the body to be constituted as an outer 'mask' for the disembodied authentic and 'youthful' inner self that creates dissonance and fractures the subjective experience of 'older'. Here cosmetic surgery is constituted as a practice for removing the 'mask' or reinscribing the materiality of the body to be commensurate with sense of self. However, rather than presenting a strategy for maintaining a 'meaningful identity' (Tulle, 2015), perhaps this discourse reveals a 'fracturing point' in discourses of ageing where 'agelessness' signifies a singularity or absence of meaning.

In *Better than Well,* Elliot (2003) identifies the dissonance between self and body as a tension in modern identity connected to enhancement technologies.

Cosmetic surgery is understood in terms of this dissonance as a practice for shaping the body in conformity with an 'inner being'. Paradoxically, what this means, as Shildrick (2008: 36) suggests, is that 'the body is viewed both as a canvas to be inscribed at will by a transcendent subject, and an integral element of selfhood'. Elliot (2003: 29) argues that the notion of an authentic self as a moral idea – 'To thine own self be true' – has 'come to suffuse contemporary life so thoroughly that we hardly recognize its presence'. This ethic, which states that 'you ought to be true to who you really are', compels individuals to find true meaning by looking inward (Elliot, 2003: 38). However, there are two problems that arise from this ethic of ageing that are central to the contention of this book. The first is that this ethic situates the body as the privileged site for ageing and the body is overinscribed by normative biomedical discourses of ageing which restrict social, cultural and subjective dimensions of ageing. The second is that the essentialist conception of the subject in this 'game of truth' is constituted as 'youthful' and 'ageless' and thus erases any conception of ageing in relation to subjectivity that might offer a critique of normative discourses of 'ageing' premised on subjective embodiment.

In order to pursue such a critique, this chapter proposes an alternative reading of 'fracture'. Following Probyn (1993), the Cartesian ethics of ageing can be viewed as the 'critical field' that renders the 'older' body and self visible and intelligible in relation to ageing. Within the context of this critical field, 'practices of the self must be positioned within the tensions of the epistemological and the ontological' (Probyn, 1993: 168). What Probyn is suggesting is that practices of self are intertwined with a problematization generated at the juncture between knowledge and subjective experience. This fracture between epistemology and ontology constitutes a point at which 'rationalization meets its limits in desubjugation' and marks 'precisely the fragility and transformability of the epistemics of power' (Butler, 2001: 15). The dissonance evidenced between self and body in relation to ageing and cosmetic surgery constitutes such a fracture. It is here, therefore that a cultural politics of 'older' can find purchase and operate to transform discourse. The remainder of the chapter engages with Foucault's theorization of subjectivation and specifically his conceptualization of the mode of subjectivation and ethical substance to explore how the 'older' self and body are rendered intelligible in ways that generate fracture.

The authentic self

Foucault (1976) described the relation of self-to-self as forming the basis for the modern hermeneutics of the subject whereby the interiority of the subject is constituted as the site for self-knowledge. Pitts-Taylor (2007: 159) argues that the culture of cosmetic surgery practice can be understood as dominated by the hermeneutics of the self – 'the culturally driven, institutionally supported need to interrogate, interpret, and assert the truth of individual subjectivity'. This 'will to self-knowledge' constitutes the mode of subjectivation to which individuals submit, not only in relation to cosmetic surgery practice, but through a vast array of contemporary practices of the self in Western societies.

In the first volume of the *History of Sexuality,* Foucault (1976) describes how the hermeneutics of the subject is linked to confessional practice as a means for telling the truth of the self that originated in Christian practice but has become widespread in social institutions including medicine and psychiatry. Foucault (1976: 61) states that the 'confession is a ritual of discourse in which the speaking subject is also the subject of the statement'. The confession is thus a technique of power and practice of subjectivation that operates to produce the self. This provides an interesting lens through which to think about the consultation between cosmetic surgeon and patient. In the context of the consultation, the patient is called upon to speak the truth of the self in relation to the appearance of the body. In this case, the authentic fixed essence of self is articulated as being incongruent with the ageing 'older' body. During the consultation confession is combined with the disciplinary technique of examination. The surgeon examines the body and provides expert judgement drawing on normative frames of reference in 'a ritual in which the truth is corroborated' (Foucault, 1976: 61). This combination provides the intersection between two powerful modes for the production of truth – the procedure of confession and medical discursivity (Foucault, 1976). During the consultation, the body is therefore offered up for scrutiny and becomes enmeshed in games of truth that govern the normative body[1] whilst the truth of the subject is generated through a hermeneutics of the self.

Foucault's work on ethics constitutes a critique of the discursive apparatus that installs the subject as an 'interiority' and psyche fixed as 'truth'. Drawing on this critique, the notion of the 'authentic youthful self' can be understood as a chimera disguising the way in which the subject is constituted through practices of self. In a lecture during his course *The Hermeneutics of the Subject*, Foucault (2005: 251) states:

> When today we see the meaning, or rather the almost total absence of meaning, given to some nonetheless very familiar expressions which continue to permeate our discourse – like getting back to oneself, freeing oneself, being oneself, being authentic, etcetera – when we see the absence of meaning and thought in all of these expressions we employ today, then I do not think we have anything to be proud of in our current efforts to reconstitute an ethic of the self.

What Foucault is suggesting is that notions of a 'true' and 'authentic' self constitute an absence of meaning. The 'authentic' self is thus a mask – not a mask of ageing – but a mask of discourse functioning as 'truth'. In other words, it is not the corporeal body that operates as a mask but the hermeneutics of the subject which masks 'the discovery that depth was only a game and surface fold' (Foucault, 1994a: 273). As Foucault (1994b: 150) elaborates:

> this is done ultimately in order to find oneself, to wrap and gather oneself in the dazzling interiority of a thought that is rightfully Being and Speech, in other words, Discourse, even if it is the silence beyond all language and the nothingness beyond all being.

If the subject remains anchored by a 'true' essence then the operation of normative modes of figuring the subject remain naturalized and taken for granted and delimit the freedom of the subject in terms of possibilities for *becoming* 'older'.

The deep interiority of the authentic self also conceals the inscription of selfhood on the materiality of the body. In cosmetic surgery discourse relating to 'older' people, the notion of an authentic self is drawn upon to justify surgery as a practice for realigning the exterior body with the interior self. However, as Blum (2003: 66) suggests:

> Surgery doesn't really seem to be about the body's interior, because the process, during which the inside becomes another outside, is ultimately topographical. There's no sense of revelation, the stunning moment of making visible what was hidden; rather there's a realignment of what constitutes the surface.

Blum's suggestion that cosmetic surgery is 'ultimately topographical' such that the 'inside becomes another outside' also constitutes a critique of the 'deep' interiority of the subject in cosmetic surgery discourse.

Extending Foucault's notion of the self, Grosz (1994: xii) draws on the metaphor of the Möbius strip to illustrate an enfolded relation between body and self:

> Bodies and minds are not two distinct substances or two kinds of attributes of a single substance but somewhere in between these two alternatives. The Möbius strip has the advantage of showing the inflection of mind into body and body into mind, the ways in which, through a kind of twisting or inversion, one side becomes another.

Through the folding of force, the outside becomes the inside establishing the interiority of the subject or 'soul'. What this conceptualization of the relation between the body and self achieves, as Grosz (1994: ix) suggests, is a 'refiguring of the body so that it moves from the periphery to the centre of analysis, so that it can now be understood as the very "stuff" of subjectivity'. She elaborates, 'All the effects of depth and interiority can be explained in terms of the inscriptions and transformations of the subject's corporeal surface' (Grosz, 1994: vii). The body conceived in this manner thus helps to problematize the dominant discourses of cosmetic surgery and ageing to view the self as constituted through practices of body modification.

Normative and deviant bodies

Drawing on Foucault's theorization of the body, Grosz (1994: 146) argues, 'the body is the field on which the play of powers, knowledges, and resistances is worked out'. As Groz (1994: 150) explains, 'discourses, made possible and exploited by power, intermesh with bodies, with the lives and behaviour of individuals, to constitute them as particular bodies'. What this means, as she elaborates, is that:

> bodies cannot be adequately understood as ahistorical, precultural, or natural objects in any simple way; they are not only inscribed, marked, engraved, by social pressures external to them but are the products, the direct effects, of the very social constitution of nature itself.
>
> (Grosz, 1994: x)

Through the inscription of norms upon the materiality and comportment of the body, bodies are rendered visible and intelligible as particular bodies. This inscription suggests that the body can be 'read' as a plane of signification, in other words as 'text', formed and given meaning within culture. In terms of 'ageing', the body is 'inescapable' (Tulle, 2015) – not just because we experience ageing as embodied subjects but because the corporeality of ageing prefigures dominant discourses of ageing.

In terms of age and cosmetic surgery practice, Charlotte feels that 'older is the time to do it more than younger because younger has the bloom of youth anyway'. Heather expresses a similar sentiment, saying 'I don't know about the young ones getting it done…Because I think that god gave them beautiful extraordinary skin. I just think their own beauty is enough'. The 'youthful' body is framed as 'god-given' and thus 'rightful' in statements such as Heather's that 'god gave them beautiful skin' and Tom's belief that younger people should not have cosmetic surgery because 'god gave you this beautiful body, wait until it is fully developed before you start mucking around with it'. The beauty of the normative body in these statements is thus constituted as 'youthful'.[2]

Dr Wilson states that older people undergo cosmetic surgery because they 'inherently want what they've lost'. That the ageing of 'older' bodies is constituted as 'loss' was also evident in an article describing cosmetic surgery for 'older' people which states 'the skin tends to hang. So the skin envelope does not tighten because they've lost so much elasticity' (Hilton, 2002). This notion of 'loss' constitutes the ageing of 'older' bodies as deviance from the normative body. In terms of 'real ageing changes', Dr Cooper states:

> So one of the arguments say for a facelift is we'll wait until you are 65 – until you see the real ageing changes and then do one operation. The other argument is to say we'll go it at 45 and you don't want to get it too bad, you don't want to look too, too bad. Do the first facelift then because you don't want to get so badly off the rails you look terrible.
>
> (Dr Cooper)

Dr Cooper's suggestion that 'ageing' can be thought as veering 'off the rails' constitutes the ageing 'older' body as deviating from the normative body.

Another way in which the 'older' body is constituted as deviant, is in texts that describe the bodies of 'older' people undergoing cosmetic surgery as requiring more extensive procedures than younger people:

> They usually require more extensive surgery, rather than limited incision and nonsurgical approaches, unless they have had plastic surgery done previously and need only maintenance procedures.
>
> (Hilton, 2002)

> Older individuals tend to need more than a mid-facelift. Typically, their aging requires correction of the forehead, face and neck.
>
> (Hilton, 2002)

> Older people are likely to need more work done because everything has aged, from the eyelids down to the neck.
>
> (Daniels, 2002)

The implication made in these statements is that greater 'correction' of ageing is needed for bodies that are significantly aged because the deviation from the idealized and 'youthful' norm is greater.

The effect of this normative rendering of the body constitutes how the body should or ought to appear and how to assign value to particular bodies. During our interview, Dr Wilson stated that 'people want to be normal, what is accepted as normal'. In cosmetic surgery discourses, 'normal' functions to produce difference as deviance whereby 'difference – even when simply age induced – signals disfigurement' (Shildrick, 2008: 35). From her interviews with women aged 24–50, Gimlin (2000: 77) argues that cosmetic surgery enables women to 'reposition their bodies as "normal" bodies' and achieve an appearance that reflects a normal self. She reports that the women in her study were not compelled to look beautiful or outstanding in any way but rather undertook cosmetic surgery 'to simply regain normal physical characteristics that they once had but had lost through the aging process' (Gimlin, 2000: 91). Correction of the changes to the body associated with ageing suggests that the aged body is examined and read according to normative standards of appearance. Normative discourses therefore inscribe deviance in the materiality of the ageing 'older' body.

In the texts generated for this book, the deviant 'older' body is pathologized through its production as 'surgically risky'. Mandy and Angela's statements amplify this theme as both expressed concerns about general anaesthetic at older ages:

> It might be more of a risk issue at an older age with anaesthetics. That would be the only thing I would be thinking about.
>
> (Mandy)

> As you get older a big anaesthetic is not good for you either, there are increased risks and infection in the hospital.
>
> (Angela)

Media texts suggested that 'special care' (Stock, 1996) and 'special precautions' (Hilton, 2002) need to be taken by surgeons operating on the bodies of older patients. The reason for the concern is the increased likelihood that older people have chronic conditions and do not heal as well as younger people:

> New surgical techniques have lessened the pain and scarring and improvements in anaesthesia and patient monitoring have made it possible to work safely on older people whose ailments had previously made them ineligible.
>
> (Stock, 1996)

> Bigger procedures in that age group like big facelifts and things are slightly more problematical because you don't heal quite as well as you get older and so, you know, there are some considerations that need to be taken, and if you have any other illnesses, you know, heart disease, that sort of thing.
>
> (Dr Smith)

Statements such as these associate the 'older' body with 'ailments' and 'illnesses' and at risk of 'perioperative complications and mortality' (Alphamaleblog, 2006). Such statements are based on epidemiological statistics that produce a positive correlation between chronological age and 'risk' for certain health problems (Mykytyn, 2008). Through this inscription of pathological decline in the materiality of the body, 'older' people are constituted as 'risky' in relation to cosmetic surgery practice.

That decline of the ageing 'older' body is normal and to be expected is evident in statements such as 'good for my age' that celebrate 'triumph' over decline (Gullette, 2004). In his interview, Tom introduces his surgeries stating 'I have had a few things done. I mean you don't get to 70 and look this good!'. In terms of health, James tells me that 'I think for my age I am quite healthy' and Heather states that whilst she is 69 she is 'a pretty fit 69 year old'. Statements such as these illustrate that biological decline of the body over time is expected and taken for granted because it is considered natural and normal (Hepworth, 2003). These statements also point to the operation of self-surveillance by 'older' people in relation to age related norms. Indeed as Cruikshank (2003: 11) observes:

> A curious pattern in gerontological research is that when questioned about their health in relation to their age, subjects tend to express a gloomy view of the health of the old in general, but consider

> themselves lucky exceptions to the decline they think characteristic of their life stage.

Cruikshank suggests that this is a 'distancing' strategy that enables 'older' people to escape stigma. Neither Cruikshank nor presumably Tom, James or Heather thought to challenge the 'truth' claims of biomedical knowledge upon the basis of subjective experience. Perhaps being healthy, fit and looking good are not states of exception to be dismissed through tropes of being 'good for one's age' but rather the grounds for a radical critique of normative discourses that constitute and delimit 'ageing' in terms of deviance and pathological decline.

The problematization of the 'ageing' of 'older' bodies is produced according to a normative assessment. This assessment reduces the 'older' body to a series of dysfunctional and deviant parts, such as sagging skin as noted earlier. To borrow from Kent's (2010: 368) writing about the fat body, in this discourse 'older' bodies are 'fragmented, medicalized, pathologized, and transformed into abject visions of the horror of flesh itself'. Drawing on Kristeva's notion of the 'abject', Kent (2010: 371) writes 'The abject sets up the categories of self and not-self, but it is an expulsion of something internal to the self.' What this suggests, in relation to the normative objectification of the 'older' body, is that the part of the body rendered deviant becomes categorized as not-self in order to be expunged. Through this process of abjection, normative discourses constitute the body as 'biomechanical' to enable reparative surgical or medical intervention undertaken by the authentic disembodied self to 'fix' the dysfunction (Shildrick, 2008).

The notion of 'fixing' the body is one that holds common currency and was evident in the interviews conducted for this study. Talking about why older people decide to have cosmetic surgery Charlotte states 'basically we want to fix our skin, that is what we want to do, all that droopy skin. Sometimes it just has to be removed because nothing but removal will fix it'. Chloe underwent liposculpture of her abdomen but was uncomfortable with the notion of facial surgery because of the association she held between her face and sense of self. She commented that, 'tummy is a different thing – a bit of tummy fat you can fix it. That's fixable'. In this statement Chloe objectifies her abdomen and constitutes her 'tummy fat' as abject. Similarly, when Tom states 'if anything starts falling, if you are 60 or 70 then get the bloody thing fixed'. The reference to body or body parts as 'thing' operates to render Tom's body 'not-self' and thus amenable to surgical intervention.

By objectifying the body, biomechanical discourses in cosmetic surgery (re)establish the Cartesian split between self and body. These discourses problematize the ageing 'older' body in terms of its deviance from the normative body. In doing so, the 'ageing' body is constituted as the ethical substance, or 'prime material of moral practice' (Foucault, 1990: 26), to be worked on using cosmetic surgery. The 'problem' is therefore not the 'older' body but the ways in which the materiality of the body is rendered governable (Dean, 1996) through its inscription by normative discourses of 'ageing'.

'New ageing': an instrument of fracture?

Within an essentialist Cartesian system of ethics, discourses of ageing problematize the appearance of the 'older' body as discordant with an 'ageless' self. This system requires problematization due to the limiting and restrictive possibilities that are afforded to subjects in terms of *becoming* 'older'. In terms of parallel identity politics, essentialist and normative systems of subjectivation have been problematized in relation to the social structuring, cultural inscription and performative enactment of identity. As Gilleard and Higgs (2013: 115) observe:

> While other visibly embodied identities such as disability, race and gender once lacked personal authority, second modernity has undermined these narratives of marginality and otherness, and women, black, gay and disabled people have acquired new forms of embodied authority enabling them to attach to their bodies more valued sources of social and cultural distinction. Age has not yet achieved this resonance.

In terms of advancing this project, Gilleard and Higgs (2013: 17) suggest that the 'new sociologies of the body' provide the discourses that might serve to reconfigure 'new ageing' in ways that recognize that 'age itself can be ambiguous or indeterminate, that it can be a site of oppression and contestation as well as an arena of choice'. These new sociologies of the body make two strategic contributions that problematize the normative, essentialist system of ageing discourses examined in this chapter. First, they work to unsettle the epistemology of 'truth' claims that install bodily 'ageing' as a 'relatively unproblematic expression of a life course that pivots naturally around a binary divide between "age" and "youth" (Gilleard and Higgs, 2013: 22). Secondly, they incite examination of the body as a site for expression of desire, performance and resistance that enables alternative possibilities for discursive inscription that might transgress the normative ageing framework. Unlike Gilleard and Higgs, however, I am more cautious about seizing discourses of 'new ageing' to advance this work. This is because, as argued in the introduction, normative discourses of 'ageing' saturated by 'truths' of corporeal decline, decrepitude and dependency have a long history of prefiguring the construction of 'older' subjectivities. Until the ontology of 'ageing' has been deeply problematized and transformed in critical scholarship, it is hazardous in its potential to reconstruct the normative boundaries that delimit possibilities for *becoming* older. Indeed the ambiguity, and thus openness, of 'becoming' as a construct of movement challenges us to think about process rather than concepts (Braidotti, 2002). As Braidotti (2002: 2) suggests, 'the point is not to know who we are, but rather what, at last, we want to become'. Braidotti's (2002: 2) perspective resonates in harmony with Foucault's in terms of understanding 'a decentred and multi-layered vision of the subject as a dynamic and changing entity' emerging from 'situated, or embedded and embodied, positions'. So rather than seize discourses of 'new ageing' with which to fracture the normative ethics of ageing, the remaining chapters dissolve the 'ageing' subject and attend to the fluid processes through which *becoming* older becomes possible and constitutes a new ethic of 'older'.

Summary

The Cartesian ethics of ageing fractures the subjective experience of 'older' in relation to the ageing of the body and sense of self. Media texts and interviewees articulate this problematization in terms of dissonance between an 'aged' appearance of the body and an internal sense of an 'ageless' self. Conceptualized in academic literature as the 'mask of ageing', this problematization constitutes an outworking of the essentialism in Cartesian ethics. This mode of ethics constitutes the critical field (Probyn, 1993) in which the 'older' body and self are rendered intelligible in relation to the practice of cosmetic surgery. In this ethical domain the self is constituted as 'authentic' through a mode of subjectivation associated with the hermeneutics of the subject. This mode of ethics constitutes the 'older' body as the ethical substance and site for ethical work. The 'older' body is problematized as declining, deviant and surgically risky through normative discourses of ageing and these discourses render features of the 'older' body abject to enable practices of surgical repair. The central contention of this chapter is therefore, that the problem is not the 'older' body but the way in which it is rendered intelligible in relation to an ethics of ageing. Thus, it is this ethics of ageing that provides the site for ethical problematization and strategic critique in order to advance a cultural politics of *becoming* 'older'.

Notes

1 Interestingly, according to Heyes and Jones (2009) contemporary movements taking place within cosmetic surgery practice are challenging the authority of the surgeon's judgement of the body. Through the outworking of consumer discourse in cosmetic surgery, surgeons are increasingly being constituted as 'service providers' rather than experts in aesthetics and required to produce results that satisfy the patient's requests or risk losing their patronage. As Heyes and Jones see it, this movement is coupled with an increasing preference for aesthetics that challenge surgeon's production of 'normal' aesthetics.
2 The problematization of 'youthful' aesthetic ideals is pursued in Chapter 4.

References

Alphamaleblog. 2006. *Cosmetic Surgery for the Elderly* [Online]. Available: www.alphamaleblog.com/cosmetic-surgery-for-the-elderly.html [Accessed 13 March 2008].

Askegaard, S., Gertsen, M. & Langer, R. 2002. The Body Consumed: Reflexivity and Cosmetic Surgery. *Psychology & Marketing*, 19, 793–812.

Blum, V. L. 2003. *Flesh Wounds: The Culture of Cosmetic Surgery*. California: University of California Press.

Braidotti, R. 2002. *Metamorphoses: Towards a Materialist Theory of Becoming*. UK & USA: Polity Press.

Butler, J. 2001. *What is Critique? An Essay on Foucault's Virtue* [Online]. Available: http://www.law.berkeley.edu/centers/kadish/what%20is%20critique%20J%20Butler.pdf [Accessed 30 August 2006].

Cruikshank, M. 2003. *Learning to be Old: Gender, Culture and Aging*. Boston: Rowman & Littlefield.

Daniels, N. 2002. So What's Wrong With Wrinkles? *The Times*.

Dean, M. 1996. Foucault, Government and the Enfolding of Authority. In: Barry, A., Osborne, T. & Rose, N. (eds) *Foucault and Political Reason: Liberalism, Neo-liberalism and Rationalities of Government*. Chicago: The University of Chicago Press.

Elliot, C. 2003. *Better than Well: American Medicine Meets the American Dream*. New York: W.W. Norton & Company.

Featherstone, M. & Hepworth, M. 1991. *The Body: Social Process and Cultural Theory*. Thousand Oaks: Sage.

Foucault, M. 1976. *The Will to Knowledge: The History of Sexuality Volume 1*. London: Penguin Books.

Foucault, M. 1990. *The Use of Pleasure: The History of Sexuality Volume 2*. USA: Vintage Books.

Foucault, M. 1994a. Nietzsche, Freud, Marx. In: Faubion, J. D. (ed.) *Michel Foucault: Aesthetics, Method and Epistemology*. New York: The New York Press.

Foucault, M. 1994b. The Thought of the Outside. In: Faubion, J. D. (ed.) *Michel Foucault: Aesthetics, Method, and Epistemology*. New York: The New Press.

Foucault, M. 1997. Subjectivity and Truth. In: Lotringer, S. & Hochroth, L. (eds) *The Politics of Truth*. USA: Semiotext(e).

Foucault, M. 2005. *The Hermeneutics of the Subject: Lectures at the College De France 1981–1982*. New York: Picador.

Gilleard, C. & Higgs, P. 2013. *Key Issues in Modern Sociology: Ageing, Corporeality and Embodiment*. London: Anthem Press.

Gimlin, D. 2000. Cosmetic Surgery: Beauty as Commodity. *Qualitative Sociology*, 23, 77–98.

Grosz, E. 1994. *Volatile Bodies: Toward a Corporeal Feminism*, Indiana: Allen & Unwin.

Grove, V. 2000. 'Under The Knife I Find The Real Me'. *The Times*, 26 February.

Gullette, M. 2004. *Aged by Culture*. Chicago: University of Chicago Press.

Hepworth, M. 2003. Ageing Bodies: Aged by Culture. In: Coupland, J. & Gwyn, R. (eds) *Discourse, the Body and Identity*. Hampshire: Palgrave Macmillan.

Heyes, C. & Jones, M. 2009. Cosmetic Surgery in the Age of Gender. In: Heyes, C. & Jones, M. (eds), *Cosmetic Surgery: A Feminist Primer*. Surrey: Ashgate Publishing.

Hilton, L. 2002. Older Americans Have Special Cosmetic Surgery Needs. *Cosmetic Surgery Times Special Reports*, 1 June.

Kaufman, S. R. 1986. *The Ageless Self: Sources of Meaning in Late Life*. Wisconsin: The University of Wisconsin Press.

Kent, L. 2010. Fighting Abjection: Representing Far Women. In: Moore, L. J. & Kosut, M. (eds) *The Body Reader*. New York & London: New York University Press.

Morton, K. 2015. Emerging Geographies of Disciplining the Ageing Body: Practising Cosmetic Technologies in the Aesthetic Clinic. *Gender, Place & Culture*, 22, 1041–1057.

Mykytyn, C. E. 2008. Medicalizing the Optimal: Anti-aging Medicine and the Quandry of Intervention. *Journal of Aging Studies*, 22, 313–321.

Öberg, P. 2003. Image versus Experience of the Aging Body. In: Faircloth, C. A. (ed.) *Aging Bodies: Images and Everyday Experience.* Walnut Creek: AltMira Press.
Pinch, E. 2008. The Rise of Silver Surgery. *Liverpool Daily Post*, 17 January.
Pitts-Taylor, V. 2007. *Surgery Junkies: Wellness and Pathology in Cosmetic Culture.* New Jersey: Rutgers University Press.
Powell, J. L. & Longino, C. F. 2002. Postmodern Versus Modernism: Rethinking Theoretical Tensions in Social Gerontology. *Journal of Aging and Identity*, 7, 219–226.
Probyn, E. 1993. *Sexing the Self: Gendered Positions in Cultural Studies.* London: Routledge.
Shildrick, M. 2008. Corporeal Cuts: Surgery and the Psycho-social. *Body & Society*, 14, 31–46.
Stock, R. W. 1996. Senior Class: Face-Lift Surgery Gains Adherents. *The New York Times*, 25 July.
The CanadianPress. 2002. More People 65 And Older Getting Cosmetic Surgery. 24 July.
Tulle-Winton, E. 2000. Old Bodies. In: Hancock, P., Hughes, B., Jagger, E., Paterson, K., Russell, R., Tulle-Winton, E. & Tyler, M. (eds) *The Body, Culture and Society: An Introduction.* Buckingham: Open University Press.
Tulle, E. 2015. Theorising Embodiment and Ageing. In: Twigg, J. & Martin, W. (eds) *Routledge Handbook of Cultural Gerontology.* Oxon & New York: Routledge.
Twigg, J. 2004. The Body, Gender, and Age: Feminist Insights in Social Gerontology. *Journal of Aging Studies*, 18, 59–73.

4 To look *better*, not younger[1]

Introduction

The discourses that inscribe the rationalities evoked in the practice of cosmetic surgery by 'older' people are explored and critically examined in this chapter. This is a significant site for analysis given Pitt's (2006: 38) insight that 'the interior meanings of cosmetic surgery are being inscribed on the bodies of people who get cosmetic surgery as much as their bodies are inscribed by their inner meanings'. Firstly, the reoccurring prefix of 're', as it is evoked in the language of rejuvenation, reversal and renewal, is examined. Through this language 'anti-ageing' discourses inscribe 'ageing' in the practice of cosmetic surgery in relation to 'older' people. Following this, anti-ageing discourses are problematized through a critique of cosmetic surgery as an ageist practice and 'older' people who undergo cosmetic surgery as denying ageing. The chapter then pursues the way in which 'older' people navigate and problematize normative anti-ageing discourses to provide an account and rationality of cosmetic surgery practice in their own terms. Here the critical impetus offered by a number of participants that cosmetic surgery is undertaken to look *better* not younger is developed to suggest that 'older' people engage with cosmetic surgery as an ethical practice of self-care. Guided by these insights, the discourses deployed in regimens of rationality shaping cosmetic surgery as it is engaged in by 'older' people are explored to argue that the forms of rationality associated with cosmetic surgery constitute a contemporary regimen of 'care of the self' in which ethical and governmental imperatives connect through the aesthetics of 'lifestyle'. This regimen provides the *tekhne* (Foucault, 2005) for exercising ethical agency and creative self-stylization. However, this analysis also recognizes that aesthetic stylization exists in the context of power relations and as such is a delimited freedom in struggles 'to both resist disciplinary power matrices and carve out a space for self-empowerment and creative choice' (Gabardi, 2001: 78). It is from this perspective that claims that cosmetic surgery is undertaken to look 'better' and not 'younger' gain a political and ethical momentum in resistance to normative discourses of 'anti-ageing'.

'Re': unbecoming and anti-ageing discourse

The prefix of 're' brings concepts such as renovation, rejuvenation, reversal, refresh, reposition, and restoration into alignment. These concepts are commonly evoked in association with the practice of cosmetic surgery by 'older' people and suggest something akin to 'putting the body back'. These are almost Mandy's words when she says, 'if you look at yourself and everything is going south, you want to put yourself back'. This notion of 're' suggests both temporal and spatial reversal of corporeal ageing:

> We are in the age of the sexy sixties and even the smoldering seventies, with a record number of older people seeking surgical assistance to beat back the ravages of time, southern drift and a face like a wrung out dishcloth.
>
> (Hamilton, 2006)

> Cosmetic plastic surgery is a safe and effective way to reverse the effects of time and gravity, according to Zenn. 'We're talking about face tissues that are beginning to sag, the eye tissues, we're talking blepharoplasty, which is a sort of eyelift, and elevating the brow or a browlift. So everything heads south, we try to move it back to north.
>
> (DukeMed News, 2005)

In these excerpts temporal reversal of ageing is suggested by beating back 'time', whilst spatial reversal of ageing is suggested by moving features of the body 'north'.

The idea that through cosmetic surgery age can be 'erased' from the appearance of the body is suggested in a media report (The Canadian Press, 2002) featuring Hazel York, an 81 year old, who 'underwent a five-hour face-lift in June in Beverly Hills, Calif., to erase some wrinkles and shave off a few years'. Similarly, Heather states that chemical peels 'will take away your age'. The idea that age can be erased to restore a relatively 'youthful' appearance is what is meant by the term rejuvenation· According to Dr Watts, patients in the 65–75 years age group are seeking facial rejuvenation to restore a youthful appearance and 'treat the signs of ageing'. Dr Williams suggests that rejuvenation entails 'Sprucing up. Spring-cleaning. Making look younger. You can do it with a piece of furniture can't you? The same with the face I think'. Here Dr Williams uses the metaphor of 'sprucing up' furniture to compare cosmetic surgery to restoration. One media text (Hilton, 2002) suggests a similar notion of renovation, suggesting that 'older' people might 'need repositioning, and perhaps a little more skin redraping'.

Rather than waiting to reverse corporeal ageing, many of the practitioners interviewed for this study emphasized prevention. Ms Robinson suggests that ageing can be prevented when she states:

> a lot of the preventative stuff that we do is mainly anti-ageing type treatments and that and educating the client, you know, it's more, 'if you do this, this and this', perhaps 'you won't look like this, this and this, in five years'.

In terms of hair loss associated with ageing, Dr Brown also proposes preventative intervention when he states:

> Because now we can avoid that look. Don't let it happen. Take some medication. Get some laser brushes onto your head and start regrowing your hair, do things to prevent that happening. Hold on to every hair you can.

Dr Smith was among others who suggested that people elect to have cosmetic surgery when they begin to associate changes to the appearance of their face with the ageing of a parent. She states, 'quite a few people who come in for upper eyelids will say "I look like my mum or dad and I've seen how they've ended up. So I don't want to go down that track"'. What this suggests is that changes to the body over time are caused by biological ageing and these changes can be prevented or reversed through the practice of cosmetic surgery.

It is useful to draw a parallel here with Murray's (2005) writing on the fat body. Through the notion of 're', the 'older' body, like the fat body, 'exists as a deviant, perverse form of embodiment and, in order to be accorded personhood, is expected to engage in a continual process of transformation, of becoming and, indeed, unbecoming' (Murray, 2005: 155). The notion of 're' and this 'unbecoming' are given meaning through anti-ageing discourses.

Mykytn (2006) suggests that anti-ageing can be considered a social movement and observes that during the past decade there has been a phenomenal growth in anti-ageing medicine. Anti-ageing medicine refers to practices, products and treatments arising from the research and development efforts of biogerontology. This discipline is dedicated to the scientific study of the biology of the ageing process (Fishman, Binstock and Lambrix, 2008). Cosmetic surgery, however, does not directly arise from developments in this discipline. As Dr Watts explained to me, anti-ageing medicine focuses on medical interventions such as 'nutritional supplementation and bio-identical hormones and things like that which are becoming more mainstream and becoming very much part of the anti-ageing movement'. He suggested that 'Surgery is probably at the perimeter of that'. Whilst cosmetic surgery can be understood as being at the disciplinary fringe of anti-ageing knowledge and development· its practice is informed by anti-ageing discourse· This link is evident in Mykytn's (2006: 644) statement that, 'Anti-ageing practitioners assert that there is much more that technoscience can do to retard, halt, and even reverse aging'.

Problematizing anti-ageing discourse

Through anti-ageing discourse, 'ageing' has become enmeshed in understanding the practice of cosmetic surgery. This discourse operates to draw a distinction between certain practices constituted as 'anti-ageing' and others which may then be considered simply aesthetic or reconstructive. In other words, through the outworking of anti-ageing discourse procedures such as facelifts, facial fat injections, neck lift and blepharoplasty (eye bag removal) are positioned as qualitatively different to rhinoplasty (nose job), octoplasty (ear pinning) and liposuction (body sculpting). This discourse enables rhinoplasty, to alter the contour of the nose, to be seen as different to having a blepharoplasty, to alter the contour of the eyes. Moreover, whilst the statement that facelifts are an 'anti-ageing' procedure is rendered intelligible by this discourse, the parallel claim that liposuction is an 'anti-fat' procedure and to undergo this procedure constitutes a denial of one's inherent 'fatness' is nonsensical. In addition, given that the purpose of anti-ageing procedures is seemingly to 'put the body back', it is interesting to consider why these procedures are not classified as reconstructive plastic surgery and funded by public health.

The distinction between practices considered 'anti-ageing' and others is being blurred through the expansion of the anti-ageing market. A UK based website (Cosmetic Surgery Consultants, 2008) on anti-ageing cosmetic surgery procedures, for example, includes liposuction amongst the listed procedures and states that 'in the realms of trying to remain looking as young and fit as possible, cosmetic surgery can work wonders'. What is suggested in this text is that looking fit, and thus presumably slender, through the use of liposuction is within the remit of 'anti-ageing'. This colonization of procedures indicates the power of anti-ageing discourse which is linked to burgeoning multi-billion dollar industries globally (Freedonia Group, 2005; Munro, 2009). The size, spread and value of this market is relevant because through anti-ageing discourse the potential market base for procedures is extended to everyone who is ageing – which is everyone.

Despite the fact that everyone is ageing and potentially a consumer of anti-ageing cosmetic procedures, in many of the texts generated for this book, the assumption that 'older' consumers of cosmetic surgery would be having 'anti-ageing' procedures operated to differentially position an 'older' consumer group in relation to 'younger' consumers. These texts produced the notion that 'younger' consumers of cosmetic surgery have procedures that alter the size, shape or contour of the body whereas 'older' consumers want to 'put the body back' and reverse the appearance of 'ageing'. Dr Watts for example' illustrates this distinction in his statement that:

> in that demographic that we are talking about – the 65–75 group – it's not that they've got thin lips that they have had all their life and they want to see what they look like plump – that's more in the 20–30 year age group where you are not dealing with age related change you are just dealing with their body as it is. And they might not like their nose or their cheeks and they might want to try something for that.

In this statement, Dr Watts suggests that unlike people in the 65–75 year old category who have undergone 'age related change', the bodies of 20–30 year olds are unaffected by ageing and so 'you are just dealing with their body as it is' which might require procedures to alter the shape of the body. So whilst 'younger' bodies have aged, because everyone is ageing, these bodies are viewed as unproblematic in terms of 'age related change' and thus not requiring 'anti-ageing' procedures.

The differentiation between age categories according to procedures is problematized by statements such as that made by Martin Kelly, a consultant plastic surgeon in the UK, and reported by The British Association of Aesthetic Plastic Surgeons (2005):

> Older patients usually ask to 'turn back the clock' – younger patients want to change their shape. But a number of senior patients have recently become more daring, and I believe largely because of the influence of happy younger patients they know, seeking to change their shape as well, having their nose done or breasts augmented.

Here Kelly suggests that 'older' consumers are becoming 'more daring' and also seeking procedures that 'change their shape' as opposed to only 'anti-ageing' procedures. Another example is provided by Dr Cooper who describes the following case:

> But one of the more interesting – patient who was in his 70s, early 70s I think and he said 'I want my ears back here', and he had these great big ears out here. I expected that, as we age our ears get stiffer, the cartilage in our ears and sometimes when you are in your 60s and 70s it is almost calcified…I reached over and they were as soft as baby's ears…He said I have spent all my life hating my ears and my wife has just died of Alzheimer's, I nursed her through that, I am at a time in my life where I want to do something for myself. And I want to know that when I lie in my coffin that I have got these ears that are pinned back. I said if you are prepared to go through it and I explained all the potential downsides, bleeding and these sorts of things, and we did it and he got a lovely outcome and he was extremely happy.

Presumably, this case was interesting because the male patient was in his seventies and wanted octoplasty (ear pinning) which is not considered an 'anti-ageing' procedure. The procedures undertaken by 'older' participants in this study included surgery for gynecomastia, liposuction, abdominoplasty, breast reduction and rhinoplasty which are not typically categorized as 'anti-ageing'. These examples suggest that the differential positioning of 'older' consumers in relation to 'younger' consumers based upon the procedures they select is unstable and tenuous. However, that anti-ageing discourse is a form of rationality 'inscribed on the bodies of people who get cosmetic surgery' as Pitts (2006: 38) suggests, becomes evident in claims that cosmetic surgery is an ageist practice and 'older' consumers are denying ageing.

In a media article titled 'More People 65 and Over Getting Cosmetic Surgery' (The Canadian Press, 2002), Leni Marshall, chairwoman of the 2002–2002

Aging and Ageism Caucus for the National Women's Studies Association, stated that cosmetic surgery 'reinforces the culture's negative view of aging'. According to 'the 32-year-old Marshall', 'People refuse to value who they've become when they get old', and 'They try and be as young as possible and plastic surgery only perpetuates it'. Similarly, in an article titled 'So What's Wrong with Wrinkles? (Daniels, 2002), Dr Merryn Gott, a lecturer in gerontology at Sheffield University, is reported to have stated that, 'Much of the problem lies with a society that doesn't value age' and 'people who buy into this ideal of youth – which is driven by the massive market in products that deny ageing, from wrinkle cream to Viagra will always be dissatisfied because the older you get, the harder it is to achieve'. These media texts draw on the authoritative voices of experts in ageing to problematize cosmetic surgery as a practice that perpetuates cultural ageism and consumers as 'buying in' to the 'pursuit of eternal youth' (Ryan, 2001) and thus denying ageing.

In media texts generated for this study, the outworking of anti-ageing discourse enabled 'older' people who undergo cosmetic surgery to be subject to disdain:

> men, by and large, go into full blown denial, continuing to delude themselves that they are permanently somewhere between 35 and 45.
>
> (Ryan, 2001)

> The 70-year-old who has restructured her face to look 50 is not to be admired and emulated but pitied.
>
> (Daniels, 2002)

These statements suggest that 'older' people who engage in cosmetic surgery are in denial, deluded and should be pitied. In our interview, James was critical of people who engage in 'anti-ageing' practices because in trying to appear 'younger' he felt they were 'living a lie'. He states:

> Film actors for instance, you know when they have had face lifts, it is just not them. They are just living a lie aren't they?...What is their aim in life? What are they trying to prove? Do they want to stay young all their lives. Their body is still growing old. We've often said, even a situation where people dye their hair when they get older, they've got an old wrinkled face, and dyed hair. It doesn't look right. An old wrinkled face should have grey hair, it's natural. I don't know whether you agree with that, but we have often said that. Even when you get older, you see a man with a big mop of hair; it doesn't always look natural, because old men very often don't have mops of hair. If that is how they are well that is how they are, but we have often said that people who dye their hair shouldn't really do that, because it doesn't look natural. I know people who do it and they do not look natural, but it is their choice. So once again they are living a lie, they are dying their hair and making themselves, trying to make themselves, look younger.

Claims such as these, that people who engage in cosmetic surgery are trying to 'stay young' and deny ageing, are enmeshed with normative ideas of how a body should appear at particular ages as though this were an unproblematic given. These normative ideas are rendered intelligible through the discourse of 'natural ageing' as James statement illustrates when he states that 'an old wrinkled face should have grey hair, it's natural'. Diversity of appearance according to 'natural ageing' is thus reduced to looking 'good for your age' or 'premature ageing'.

This reductive reading of the body, in which 'age' operates to norm appearance, retains a latent essentialism premised upon the constitution of the 'naturally ageing body'.[2] Interestingly, an alternative reading of cosmetic surgery that evades this essentialism is offered by anti-ageing discourse. As Mykytyn (2006: 644) states, anti-ageing discourse 'bypasses the construct of aging as natural or a disease, for the goal of optimizing health and bodily experience'. What this notion of bypassing ageing suggests is that rather than denying ageing by attempting to appear 'younger', cosmetic surgery can be understood as aesthetic enhancement to optimize health and bodily experience.

Aesthetic enhancement: To look better not younger

Charlotte, Sophie, Emily, Tom, Chloe, and Mandy all suggest that cosmetic surgery is practiced to enhance appearance and in doing so feel better. In Tom's words, 'I just want to look good. I like to look good' and 'because I feel I look good, I feel good'. Charlotte states, 'I didn't want to look younger than people that are younger than me, I just wanted to look still like me, but I wanted to get rid of – and it did disappear – the droopy, the lines, the area that has been refreshed'. In relation to surgical techniques for the face, Dr Wilson states, 'we're optimising it to look younger, to look better. To look better. Optimise. Whatever it is there, optimise'. What these extracts suggest is that relative improvement – feeling and looking better – is what is important. As Dr Wilson suggests 'we all choose to look younger. Why do we choose to look younger? Not because we want to look younger but because we want to look better. If you think about it. We don't want to look younger, we want to look better'. He states 'It's not like "Oh I'm putting your face back, this is now ten years would you like twenty? Okay that's there". It doesn't work that way. But we're optimising it to look better and so whilst 'people say "Hey turn back ten years". You know, that's a perception'. These extracts from my interview with Dr Wilson problematize the association between cosmetic surgery and anti-ageing discourse because they begin to suggest that the practice of cosmetic surgery is not literally about rewinding the chronological clock but improving the aesthetic appearance of the face without needing to evoke age. His suggestion that the reversal of 'age' is just a perception speaks to the impossibility of actually reversing ageing and the operation of age norms in judgments of appearance. This allows us to consider whether 'anti-ageing' procedures are ultimately any different from other procedures used to change body size, shape or contour given that the rationality informing the practice of all cosmetic procedures is aesthetic enhancement.

Jones (2004: 528) argues that 'the aim of cosmetic surgery is to make people look "better, not younger"'. She elaborates that 'contrary to appearances, it is less about reclaiming or reinventing youthfulness and more about attempting to create a look of indeterminate age or "agelessness"' (Jones, 2004: 527). In conclusion, Jones (2004: 527) states that cosmetic surgery allows 'people to control the aesthetics of their ageing process'. This point is also made by Gilleard and Higgs (2000: 132–133) who suggest that:

> In the absence of an inner logic to ageing, the play of signification that is involved in choosing how and when to age offers a wide scope for the marketing of desire. Skin peels, tummy tucks, forehead lifts, hair transplants, botox injections and facial fat grafting do not 'restore' a youthful appearance so much as improve the 'aesthetic' appearance of the ageing face. To that extent cosmetic surgery is less about anti-ageing and more to do with a general desire felt by many to improve upon their 'natural' appearance.

Gilleard and Higgs reject the concept of a 'naturally ageing body' through their suggestion that there is an 'absence of an inner logic to ageing'. They also suggest the potential for a 'play of signification' writ large in the materiality of the 'older' body. This play of signification entails 'aesthetics' and improved appearance. Such aesthetic concerns, as Pitts-Taylor (2009: 126) suggests, matter, in that they are 'deeply superficial, with all of the contradictions that term might imply'. This distinction between looking younger and looking better is thus one of great significance for the cultural politics of 'older'.

In terms of contemporary cultural understandings of aesthetics, looking 'good' has become profoundly conditioned by notions of 'youthfulness' whilst looking 'better' is deeply enmeshed with notions of looking 'younger'. In this way 'ageing' norms 'extend their own power to order the entire field of moral and political judgment' concerning the appearance of the body (Butler, 2001: n.p.). From the standpoint that practices of self-care constitute a form of critique, the distinction made by 'older' participants that cosmetic surgery is about looking *better* rather than looking younger can be interpreted as a means of influencing the rationality that informs engagement with cosmetic surgery. This entails an act of resistance to anti-ageing discourse and oppressive interpretations that to undergo cosmetic surgery is to deny ageing and perpetuate ageist practices. Acts of resistance are also acts of freedom to achieve a desirable mode of being (Foucault, 1994). This calls for an exploration of the ethos that shapes 'older' people's engagement with cosmetic surgery.

Care of self and lifestyle

In our interview Chloe makes connections between appearance, lifestyle and symbolic status[3] when she states:

> I think appearance has become very important in all our lifestyles. If you're young, ambitious, climbing the ladder, male or female, your appearance is actually very very important. That goes along with the fashion, the labels you wear, the car you drive, the whole thing is status. There's a status symbol in there as well because you want the best. You want the ultimate. We are all driven to have the latest car, the latest flat screen TV, the new kitchen, we work for lifestyle.

She goes on to suggest that at present cosmetic surgery practice is a part of lifestyle saying, 'I think we accept it more, we see it as part of a lifestyle in a lot of ways. Going back 50 years I don't think my parents would have thought of cosmetic surgery, it wouldn't have been available to them unless it was for a medical reason'. These extracts from Chloe's interview speak to the notion that in contemporary neoliberal consumer society, the ethical subject is compelled to provide style to life and personal identity through practices of consumption and that cosmetic surgery is embedded in this ethos. Here, 'lifestyle' is linked to an art of existence and rationalities 'of the government of oneself' (Foucault, 1990: 89) that constitute a contemporary regimen of self-care. In the discussion to follow, the rationalities inscribed in cosmetic surgery are elaborated in relation to a regimen of self-care. This discussion situates cosmetic surgery as a technology discursively positioned at the nexus between aesthetic enhancement, therapeutic intervention and consumer choice. In doing so, this chapter unfolds a regimen of rationality that establishes cosmetic surgery as a practice of self: as an enhancement technology cosmetic surgery is associated with self-improvement; as a therapeutic intervention it is associated with self-fulfilment; and, as a consumable it is associated with self-indulgence.

Self-care: bodily maintenance

Once considered socially and culturally undesirable and associated with superficiality and vanity, 'body work' to enhance appearance has undergone a discursive transformation into ethical self-care. Through the course of this research I became aware that the notion of 'vanity' was rarely evoked but when it was, it had evidently become grafted to socially and culturally acceptable ideas of 'looking after yourself'. Chloe, Mandy and Heather problematized vanity in similar terms stating:

> Vain people are often very precious and far too preoccupied with their own looks and appearance. I don't think that is a good thing, I wouldn't like to be labelled vain. But vanity does mean caring about how you look and making the best of what you have got to face the world.
>
> (Chloe)

> My daughter says I am vain and I suppose I am because I just want to make the best of what I have got…I haven't thought of myself as vain. I

> have always done my hair and put makeup on every day, I can't not do that. I always have.
>
> (Mandy)

> Well if I am going out I want to look the best I can look. It's like someone gets a facelift then that's the best they can. So, I am not going to get a face-lift, I'm going to put my make-up on and brighten my face…And I suppose if that's vanity then I am vain. But it's more routine, I have always done it.
>
> (Heather)

In our interview I drew Dr Watts' attention to the receding notion of vanity and he responded that:

> People do, patients do sort of say I know it's being vain but I am worried about this or that. So, I do think that they feel some embarrassment about seeking advice on a particular problem that troubles them. I mean what is vanity? I think everyone is vain if you define it as wanting to look better and all being concerned about your appearance. Or else we wouldn't wear clothes and get our hair cut and brush our teeth.

These statements suggest that cosmetic surgery to 'look better' belongs to a regimen of self-care concerning appearance that is routine.

Many of the participants interviewed in this study suggested that body practices including cosmetic surgery are part of a regimen of ongoing labour for maintaining the body. According to Ms Robinson, cosmetic surgery once you are 'older' is 'too late really, for a lot of people, because they take their skin for granted when they are young and don't maintain what they are born with really. They neglect it'. According to the studied texts, maintenance of the body needs to begin as early as possible and, as illustrated by Chloe's and Charlotte's statements, is an ongoing commitment:

> My personal maintenance, in my business I feel a certain pressure, and especially at my age it is harder and harder to look good and present well in your clothes, face, hair, the whole package. I do spend a bit on maintenance including hair colour which I think is the biggest give away to age, your greying hair. So I do spend money maintaining my hair. I am very conscious of my skin and cleaning, toning and all the rest of those procedures that we women do.
>
> (Chloe)

> What I decided was before the lines get deeper, before they get deeper, looking and thinking if I do it now it won't show. I have one friend in the time I have known her, she has had two face lifts and she has a lovely face but you have to maintain it, you still have to work on it.
>
> (Charlotte)

Tom draws a parallel between maintenance of the body and maintenance of a car in his comment that 'if your car breaks down you get it fixed, if the paint goes off you want to get it sprayed or get a new one. You can't get a new one of these but you can fix it' (also see Chapter 3).

Chloe, Mandy, Angela and Tom consider this body work 'taking care of themselves'. The reverse of this, as Dr Smith and Dr Wilson suggest, are individuals who do not engage in ongoing body work and have 'let themselves go'. According to this perspective, cosmetic surgery is positioned as no different to other cosmetic procedures for maintaining and enhancing appearance:

> Jenny, mid 70s. Had a facelift 20 years ago, and has just had her brow lifted and work done around her eyes. I think if people want anything done, they should go ahead. What's the difference? We all like to look our best. Is there any difference between this and going to the dentist or the hairdresser?
>
> (Linnell, 1999)

> I mean we buy new clothes, don't we, to look good. We try to look the best we can when we go out. It's not always to attract a man. It's just so you like yourself and think you look the best you can, you know. So therefore I find that if you are going to buy a new suit then why not. I mean you get your nails done and you get your feet done, what's the difference? It all comes under cosmetic.
>
> (Heather)

> You know, you want to look good and feel good so you get your hair done so you want to look good and feel good so you go and see if you, you know, can have your crows feet done. I don't see there's a lot of difference between the two.
>
> (Dr Williams)

As these statements suggest, cosmetic surgery is becoming increasingly normalized as a practice of care of the self.

The empirical texts collectively suggested that the acceptance and popularity of cosmetic surgery as a means for 'taking care of oneself' is rising in relation to increasing affordability and safety and reduction in invasiveness and 'down time':

> 'Cosmetic surgery has become more acceptable and financially it has become more affordable. Our mothers might have gone to Tupperwear parties but this generation is more likely to be invited to Botox parties', Martell said. With wrinkle-buster botox now considered mainstream, Martell's tip for the next beauty trend was fat-removing liposuction in your lunch break.
>
> (Online, 2006)

Reflecting on the increasing popularity and normalization of cosmetic surgery, Dr Williams states: 'It used to be unnecessary, the rich and famous, the Hollywood sector…Now it's more: It's safe, it's affordable, why not, I feel better about myself, everybody's doing it'. When I asked Dr Williams whether he thought older people having cosmetic surgery is just part of that wider societal increase in cosmetic surgery he replied 'Yes' I do' and it's more affordable'.

In terms of a regimen of self-care, Tom spoke about many of the practices he uses to take care of his body and appearance including maintaining a low fat diet, exercising, drinking alcohol in moderation, never smoking and skin care.

> Exercise, I like to exercise. I think for my age I have kept pretty well. Though I don't look it I am very muscly. I am pretty good actually for my age. Like I said, I do look after myself food wise, I'm not a drinker. Don't get me wrong I do drink but I'm not a drinker.

> It's probably because I know a lot of 70 year olds who aren't all as good as me, can't look as good as me. But then you have got to take things into consideration. I have got a sister four down and she looks 10 years older than me. Not just now [after cosmetic surgery] but even the way I was. She is a smoker – very heavy. I have never smoked.

> I put lots of sunscreen on when I go out in the sun. I have lots of cosmetic cream but I don't advertise that. When I say cosmetic cream it's not me. That L'Oreal I put it on. Why not, it looks after your skin.

In three of these excerpts Tom evokes his chronological age in relation to his appearance to suggest that through taking care of himself he has maintained an appearance that is 'good for his age'. As Chapter 1 asserts, such statements are conditional on and reinstate the norms that govern judgement of the appearance of ageing. Similarly, when I probed Angela as to why she thought certain people do not look their age she responded that 'lots of them do look after themselves. Years ago a lot of older people didn't, but there are a lot more things available now'. In terms of herself, she states, 'I use Nivea Q10, I don't wear a lot of make-up but simple things like that, for years I used that Oil of Ulay. People say to me you don't look that old, because my skin is not that wrinkly, it is getting more wrinkly but it is not that bad at my age'. Statements such as these open up space to question 'ageing' in terms of 'natural' bodily changes and suggest contingency in relation to environmental damage and maintenance regimen.

Cardona (2008) has explored the nexus between the ethical domain and 'anti-ageing' technologies in her research which identified 'the notion that through 'anti-ageing medicine individuals were exercising a proper care of the self' (Cardona, 2008: 478). On the basis of widespread cosmetic practices for 'taking care of the self', Gilleard and Higgs (2000: 69) argue that grey hair, sagging skin or wrinkles 'become as much a sign of personal neglect or transient weariness as an intrinsic feature of ageing'. I asked Dr Wilson if he considered appearing 'older' as largely a matter of choice and he responded at length:

> It certainly is a choice, I mean you can control elements of it. It is something that if you have been taking care of yourself since you were younger, it's a choice you have already made. It's not a choice that you can make when you're older and you've done all the wrong things, you know and you smoke all your life, you've sunned yourself…But if somebody takes care of themselves, they make the choice very early in life that they're going to take care of themselves then yeah it's a choice that they've made but it might not be surgery – just by lifestyle choices, what they eat, how they train, how they think, you know, that sort of thing. How they live, how they live their life. Because you know, how you live your life is very important.

This statement illustrates that taking care of yourself through 'good' lifestyle practices such as limiting exposure to the sun, dietary choices and exercise throughout life is an ethical commitment. The body then becomes the surface of inscription for the choices one makes and can be read in terms of its virtue. Looking 'good' or an attractive appearance thus signifies the ethical subject at all ages and stages of the life course.

The virtues associated with practices of self-care mean they are undertaken in the pursuit of happiness. As Öberg (2003: 104) suggests, we are

> constantly reminded that individuals who work to take care of their bodies stay healthier, live longer, maintain their figure, and in general, look "good". Television, film and other visual media remind us that the slim and graceful body, with dimples in the attractive face, is the key to happiness – maybe even its essence.

Here, Öberg speaks to the way in which practices to maintain and enhance corporeal experience are undertaken within the widening parameters of 'health'. According to the parameters set by the World Health Organization (1948), health is no longer a state constituted by the absence of disease but characterized by complete physical, mental and social well-being. In 1980 Crawford published his seminal article on 'healthism' in which he argued that health was becoming a 'super value' that 'subsumes a panopoly of values' including 'a sense of happiness and purpose', 'a high level of self-esteem', 'work satisfaction', 'ability to engage in creative expression' and so on and so forth. Crawford (1980: 381) suggests that:

> Less a means towards the achievement of other fundamental values, health takes on the quality of an end in itself. Good living is reduced to a

> health problem, just as health is expanded to include all that is good in life.

Citing a talk by Ardell, Crawford (1980: 380) writes, 'In the "high level wellness" ethic, "health is freedom in the truest sense – freedom from aimlessness, being able to express emotions freely, a zest for living"'. The notion that healthism provides 'freedom from aimlessness' suggests the virtue of having something to strive for. Following Foucault, Higgs and his colleagues (2009: 689) have termed this ethical imperative the 'will to health' to suggest that 'Health has become a fundamental and required goal of the individual'. As Gilleard and Higgs (2000: 9) elaborate:

> Nearly all age groups view health as the most important attribute in life. This widespread concern with improving health and personal wellbeing is reflected in an ever-widening participation in personal exercise, greater attention to diet and weight, the selective consumption of 'health' foods, vitamins and mineral supplements and the active exploration of self-expression.

This statement suggests that the 'will to health' supports active participation in the consumption of products and practices for cultivating the body and self-expression. As Rose (2001) observes, as the idea of health is reconfigured to encode an 'optimization' of an individual's corporeality, the new 'ethnopolitics' arising from somatic ethics compels the individual to improve oneself. This regimen of self-care thus becomes a lifelong commitment in which the ethical subject strives towards enhanced health and wellbeing.

The preceding discussion suggested that through a broadening conception of 'health', cosmetic surgery is becoming grafted to a socially, culturally and ethically acceptable regimen of self-care and thus increasingly freed from the stigma associated with vanity. However, cosmetic surgery retains its ambivalent position with respect to mainstream health. This is because, as a later paper by Crawford (2006: 403) attests, 'the meaningful practice of health is inextricably linked to the science, practice and layered meanings of biomedicine'. Given that cosmetic surgery constitutes an intervention for physically healthy bodies, its practice seemingly violates the Hippocratic oath and goes against 'the medical profession's fundamental principles' (Haiken, 1997: 93). The result is that 'Cosmetic surgery bears a peculiar burden of justification unlike other medical subspecialties' (Heyes, 2007: 90).

In terms of healthcare practice, Dr Brown captures the disciplinary ramifications associated with surgery for aesthetic enhancement in his statement that, 'cosmetic surgery is breaking away into a new field where we have patients who are not sick. They are well but we want to make them more well'. As this statement suggests, cosmetic surgery can be demarcated from other surgical practice on the grounds that it is elective and undertaken for aesthetic enhancement to make patients 'more well'. In his book *Better than*

Well, Elliot (2003) traces contemporary concerns and debates surrounding enhancement technologies. In his approach to this subject, Elliot (2003: xvii) draws attention to, and deliberately blurs, the boundaries constructed between 'proper medicine' and 'enhancement technologies'. As Elliot (2003: 107) explains, 'Most of what are commonly called enhancement technologies today can also be described as treatments. Viagra can enhance sexuality or treat impotence; plastic surgery can enhance the body or treat disfigurements'. As Rose (2007: 17) suggests 'The old lines between treatment, correction, and enhancement can no longer be sustained'.

The blurring of boundaries between what constitutes cosmetic and medical intervention was evident when I asked Ms Martin what she meant by the term 'cosmetic surgery' and she responded:

> Anything that's not like medical but it's like cosmetic. It is something that enhances you as a person but then, having said that, there's things like breast reductions and you know, a patient who has had a stroke whose having a facelift. That's not, I wouldn't class that as cosmetic...I mean Medicare covers it. Private health will cover it. And I mean the patient can't help they had a stroke – of course they're going to try and help them to be normal again.

As this excerpt illustrates, it is the distinction between what is considered 'normal' and 'optimal' that polarizes medical and enhancement technologies. This distinction plays out in the field of surgery to differentiate cosmetic from plastic surgery. For Dr Cooper, a plastic surgeon, 'the original description of cranial facial surgical techniques is really about treating deformity and trying to make it more normal'. Ms Martin's response also alludes to the control and policing of the boundary between the use of technologies deemed 'treatments' and those deemed 'enhancement' through public healthcare policy. Medically necessary treatments are funded whilst elective enhancement is not (Elliot, 2003). In Australia, 'non-therapeutic' cosmetic surgery procedures are not classified with an item code in the Medicare Benefits Schedule (MBS) and must be privately funded. Configuration as an enhancement technology therefore situates cosmetic surgery in an ambivalent position with respect to 'proper medicine' in that it cannot be legitimated by biomedical discourse.

The key to the discursive frames used to legitimate cosmetic surgery practice is to be found in the definition of cosmetic surgery by the Health Care Complaints Commission (HCCC). This definition states that, 'A central characteristic of cosmetic surgery is that it is initiated by the consumer to improve their appearance and self-esteem' (Health Care Complaints Commission, 1999: 4). According to this definition the 'consumer' elects to undergo cosmetic surgery to improve 'self-esteem' by improving their appearance. Cosmetic surgery practice thus 'joins the presumption of consumer rights with psychotherapeutic imperatives' (Frank, 2002: 18). Discourses that legitimate cosmetic surgery practice are therefore drawn from the frames of consumer culture and 'psy' discourses (Rose, 1996). The strategic imperative in the deployment of these discourses is to shift the focus from the 'healthy' body to the needs and desires of the self.

Self-fulfilment: the constitution of cosmetic surgery by 'psy' discourses

In the textual data cosmetic surgery was consistently associated with psychological constructs and mental health. The following extract taken from my interview with Dr Brown relates cosmetic surgery to psychological health and ability to function in society:

> There are people who genuinely do not like a particular aspect of their appearance and it becomes a focus of their attention to the point where it destabilizes their thinking processes and their ability to socialize and be a normal part of society. There's a saying in the hair restoration field that baldness is not fatal or life threatening but it is social life threatening and there are especially young people and ladies who lose hair who do become psychiatric with the condition, they withdraw from society, withdraw from work, don't want to be seen. They're depressed. What sort of outcome is that? If there's a procedure that can help them, which is safe, done well, results are pretty much what we expect, that's cosmetic surgery.

In this statement cosmetic surgery is positioned as a 'treatment' to cure or prevent depression and psychiatric symptoms that can manifest from distress and suffering associated with physical appearance. More often, however, cosmetic surgery was positioned in terms of psychological enhancement. Chris for example, states that 'cosmetic surgery is enhancement of your looks and mental health' whilst Angela suggests that although liposuction removed the 'bumps...Psychologically it was good too'. Charlotte and Chloe both reported that they specifically experienced an increase in 'confidence' following their cosmetic surgery. One media report (Grove, 2000) suggests, 'There is a real psychological advantage in confidence and appearance' and another (Media Monitors, 2007) found that '90% of patients report that they have an increased sense of self-esteem. And the word that repeatedly comes out in these surveys is increased confidence'. Enhanced confidence and self-esteem essentially mean feeling good about yourself and thus relate to an experience of subjective wellbeing. When asked whether she considers cosmetic surgery healthcare, Ms Robinson responded:

> Their mental health, their mental wellbeing. You know, the mental affects the physical, doesn't it? And how you feel about yourself, yeah, I do consider it health care for that reason, really, you know? I mean here what we're about, even though it's cosmetic, like a lot of it's cosmetic and beauty orientated, it is about the wellbeing, it is about nurturing the soul.

In this statement Ms Robinson suggests that cosmetic surgery is about nurturing the soul to achieve subjective wellbeing. As Elliot (2003: 52–53) observes:

> As our culture has shifted the locus of meaning in life away from God and onto individual psychology, we have created a moral yardstick that measures the success of a human life in terms of psychological well-being…Today, enhancement technologies are not just instruments for self-improvement, or even self-transformation – they are tools for working on the soul.

As a practice, cosmetic surgery thus assumes a therapeutic function through its constitution by 'psy' discourses (Rose, 1996).

During the development of cosmetic surgery, knowledge from the 'psy' disciplines, including psychology, psychiatry and psychoanalysis, infused its practice to legitimate surgical intervention in otherwise healthy bodies. In her book *Venus Envy,* Haiken (1997) describes the ethical dilemmas generated by 'beauty doctors' during the early development of cosmetic surgery. At this time, as it is today, the nexus between surgical intervention and aesthetic enhancement was problematized. The partial resolution of these ethical dilemmas occurred through the introduction of the 'inferiority complex' developed by the psychologist Alfred Adler. The inferiority complex, Adler argued, resulted from an individual developing a sense of personal inferiority due to physical deficiencies (Elliot, 2003). The inferiority complex therefore constituted the justification for cosmetic surgery to treat this psychological condition. As Elliot (2003: 120) observes, with the infusion of psy, 'Cosmetic surgery was successfully transformed from enhancement to treatments during the early part of the twentieth century.'

Commonly referred to as 'psychiatry with a scalpel', the regimen of rationality associated with cosmetic surgery practice now extends well beyond beauty ideals. As Pitts (2006: 40) elaborates, the dominant logics 'depend upon essentialist notions of authentic inner selves. They require an understanding of the body and its surface as a signifier of authentic inner meaning, and they recruit psychiatric strategies to decode the meanings they want to find.'

The psychiatric strategies that Pitts refers to in this quotation includes the deployment of 'psy' discourses to constitute the essential authentic self and the technique of confession used to diagnose its psychical qualities (see Chapter 3). At present, cosmetic surgery forms part of what Elliot (2003: 206) refers to as the 'therapeutic turn' whereby 'life's purpose is to develop, sustain, and fine tune psychological wellbeing'. In this context, as Pitts (2006: 38) points out, body modification practices such as cosmetic surgery have become 'a primary mode for articulating the authentic, healthy and happy self'.[4]

Self-indulgence: the constitution of cosmetic surgery by consumer discourses

The definition of cosmetic surgery from the HCCC cited previously explicitly positions people who undergo cosmetic surgery as 'consumers'. That interviewees in this study also thought of cosmetic surgery as a consumer practice was evident in statements such as Chloe's:

> You don't have to go to your doctor and say I want this problem fixed, you can go straight to your surgeon who is the specialist in that cosmetic area and say I need this done, what will it cost me and when can I get there? It is a business, a business contract between you and a specialist. You are buying that service and it is available, easily available. If you need that service and you have the money, there is nothing stopping it.

When I asked Ms Taylor whether she sees cosmetic surgery as a consumer choice she replied 'Very much so. Yeah. Like buying a car'. Dr Watts explicitly locates cosmetic surgery as a commodity in his statement that:

> If there is $10,000 for some sort of major surgical procedure, that was the cost of a television. You wouldn't even buy a used car for that, so people were used to large sums of money for houses, cars, whitegoods, kitchens and so this became pricewise a consumer commodity item.

Similarly, Dr Brown suggests that cosmetic surgery is a choice among other commodities in his statement that 'there are some people who struggle with a concept of "am I doing the right thing? Am I wasting these resources on me? We could renovate the home or buy a new car instead". But decreasingly so'.

As a commodity, cosmetic surgery is positioned in terms of a marketplace and consumer demand as illustrated by Dr Watts' suggestion that 'I think what happens in this market is that there are lots of different products and services on offer and the patients will decide on what is going to be popular and what's not'. Similarly, Dr Brown suggests that:

> cosmetic medicine and surgery is a relationship between the doctor and the patient, with no third person providing anything. And we like that. We like that because we call the tune or, at least, the consumer or patient calls the tune and if we as providers aren't up to speed with our interpersonal skills and our treatments, we will soon be discarded by the patient who is actually paying good money for our service.

In this excerpt Dr Brown suggests that cosmetic surgery is a commercial venture and that surgeons need to be competitive in the marketplace in terms of their customer service and commodities for sale if they are to attract consumer funds. Consumer discourse thus constitutes cosmetic surgery as a commodity and positions patients with agency as consumers.

The exercise of freedom in consumer societies operates through choice as an individual right, 'the right of each to spend his or her own resources as he or she chooses' (Frank, 2002: 19). Ms Taylor, who works in a plastic surgery practice with surgeons who also provide cosmetic surgery, expressed the opinion that 'it's a little bit frivolous, the additional stuff but people have got a right to spend their money where they want. It's not for me to tell them whether they should or shouldn't'. Consumer discourse thus constitutes cosmetic surgery practice as the individual right of an autonomous, freely choosing subject. Sophie asserts that 'I was doing it for myself' and similarly Tom states that 'It's how I want to look, how I want to feel'. Mandy countered the external censure from her son and daughter with the argument that 'I'd do it because I wanted to do it, and how I feel – which is the big thing'.

Dr Smith suggested that despite popular opinion women do not undertake cosmetic surgery for their partner or to attract a partner. She asserts that:

> They do it for themselves generally and women have their own money and their own abilities to do such things and I'll say to them, next time, well you know, "What did Fred think?" "Oh he didn't notice". I think mainly they do it for themselves and other women [who notice and appreciate aesthetics].

Similarly, Ms Harris stated that:

> I don't think a lot of women in my experience do any of my procedures for their partners or to attract a partner. Yeah a lot of them kind of come in and they're like "Finally". Like they've just been wanting to have it done for ages and they've never gotten around to doing something for themselves and they're just so thrilled to have it done. They're so excited. It's really good.

As this excerpt suggests, 'doing something for yourself' is a source of excitement and pleasure. Featherstone (2007: 83) observes that 'consumer goods become associated with luxury'. Chloe certainly considers cosmetic surgery a luxury as she states 'It's sort of a self-indulgence isn't it? Like buying fabulous jewellery or something. It is an indulgence.'

The association between body work and pleasure is evident in the increasing colonization of the field of cosmetic surgery by 'leisure services'. Increasingly non-invasive procedures are enabling cosmetic surgery practice to move into this social and cultural space. What this means for example, is that the practice of cosmetic surgery is physically shifting from hospitals to day clinics and consulting rooms. Cosmetic surgery clinics are often hybrid spaces (also see Morton, 2015) created at the discursive juncture between clinical environment and aesthetic space. One of the consulting rooms I visited retained the structural layout of a typical General Practice but combined these clinical features with fashionable contemporary colour schemes, plants, and the display of art work. Cosmetic procedures are also increasingly being delivered by general practitioners, nurses and beauty therapists rather than surgeons. Interestingly, one of the cosmic surgeons whose patients I interviewed had previously operated as a General Practitioner and when he moved into cosmetic surgery retained the same premises and many of his patients. The colonization of cosmetic practices by pleasure and leisure was most evident however, in my interview with Ms Robinson. When describing her business she states:

> We're a beauty clinic, cosmetic clinic. We do everything from waxing, basic waxing treatments, manicures, pedicures, day spa, warm therapies. We do IPL, photo rejuvenation, laser hair removal. We have a visiting nurse who comes in and does Botox and any fillers, that type of thing. So really we're a one stop shop.

What is interesting here is that cosmetic medicine such as Botox, fillers and laser hair removal are offered together with waxing, manicures and pedicures. In terms of this combination she says:

> You know, in the treatment rather than just going and having an injectable done. You know, we will combine their injectables with other things…We might do peels and things like that which a lot of, I think, cosmetic surgeons or surgeries don't offer in the same manner. They offer it, but differently. Not in the same sort of relaxing way that a clinic like this does. So you are taking care of their whole wellbeing.

Ms Robinson suggests that having cosmetic procedures 'not only offers the client a visual effect or a visible effect but also gives them the relaxation that gives them that bit of time out'.

Arguably the most striking example of the blending of cosmetic surgery with leisure however, is the burgeoning cosmetic surgery travel industry or 'medical tourism' (see Bell et al., 2011; Holliday et al., 2015). In this industry, flights and accommodation are 'packaged' together with surgery fees to provide consumers with cheaper surgery than at home and the opportunity to enjoy their 'down time' in exotic locations. In a newspaper article on cosmetic surgery tourism and 'mummy makeovers'' Nash (2009) writes:

> Destiny MediTravel offers a range of customised overseas surgical holiday packages for less than the price of breast implants in Australia. From about $11,000 post-baby mums can have breast augmentation and a tummy tuck, including return airfares and 14 nights accommodation in a resort in Phuket. Gorgeous Getaways, another medical travel agency, even provides the option of 24-hour babysitting for patients with young children.

Through consumer discourse cosmetic surgery is therefore constituted as a financial option and choice associated with pleasurable and indulgent practices of self.

Self-care: An ethic of creativity and freedom

Following Baudrillard, Besley and Peters (2007: 45) assert that

> in the postmodern world, the aesthetics of existence are inexorably linked with the commodification of our world and existence. Our relationship to commodities and the self is no longer based on 'need', but more on a desire that can never be satisfied so we seek new objects to consume in a system where choices are infinite, and desire and pleasure become integral parts of the material and social production that in turn produce or construct more desire/pleasure.

As this quotation suggests, the evocation of desire by a system of material and social production in which choices are infinite drives ethical projects to stylize personal identity. Desire and desirability therefore infuse socially and culturally constituted practices of self and forms of embodied subjectivity. Through these practices of self, individuals transform themselves into ethical subjects whose lives are characterized by certain aesthetic values and stylistic criteria. This implies a creative self-fashioning whereby 'subjects come to identify with some preferred version of who they want to be' (Frank and Jones, 2003: 182).

As a practice of self-care, cosmetic surgery is governed by an aesthetic and creative sensibility. That artistry is foundational to the constitution of cosmetic surgery practice, is evident in the insignia of The Australasian College of Cosmetic Surgery which promotes professional values of 'Artistry, Integrity, Excellence'. Similarly advertisements from the Feb–April 2007 edition of the Cosmetic Surgery Magazine incorporate slogans such as 'Where artistry and surgery meet' and 'Cosmetic surgery: The perfect blend of art and science'. According to Dr Brown, as a field of surgical practice, cosmetic surgery 'attracts people with artistic talent, because it allows practitioners to express that talent rather than taking out one appendix after the other'. The notion of cosmetic surgeon as artist or sculptor was particularly evident in my interview with Dr Wilson. He described cosmetic enhancement using surgery as a matter of 'fine tuning the angle of the lip' or being able to 'optimise a brow angle'. When I asked him how the art and practice of cosmetic surgery is taught he responded:

> it's very advanced training where you are taught the more refined art of surgery with regards to cosmetic purposes, so you know, it's less formulas and things like that, it's you know less formulaic surgery, it's more of a true aesthetic sort of thing where you really need to have an eye for detail, you really need to have an eye for what is beautiful, what will make a person look good.

I pressed him further to explain how they teach surgeons what is aesthetically pleasing and he suggested that 'a good cosmetic surgeon is basically born with that eye'. Having an 'eye' for aesthetics positions the surgeon as having innate artistic sensibilities. He went on to state:

> It is an art, I mean that's the thing, there's no formulas that fits it proper…I'm also very good with breast implants and things like that but where I have a knack of knowing how much and how to tilt the tissues but when it comes to a breast lift I don't have the algorithm in my head.

Cosmetic surgery as an 'art' requiring the 'knack' or 'know-how' constitutes the surgeon as an expert craftsman in aesthetics of the body.

The blurring of boundaries between surgery and art by cosmetic surgeons has been taken to new levels by surgeons who engage in traditional forms of art. Jones (2008: 72) observes that, 'the most surprising change for me since 1998 is the propensity of cosmetic surgeons who now display their own works of art. It seems that cosmetic surgeons are also painters, photographers, sculptors and even musicians'. One example is Sydney cosmetic Surgeon Dr Anoop Rastogi. An article (Alexander, 2007) in the *Cosmetic Surgery Magazine*, reports Dr Rastogi's art exhibition and new book *Breast Art: A Fusion of Art and Surgery*, both of which feature photographic images of actual patients. Dr Rastogi is reported to have stated:

> with the artistic skill to visualise a breast sculpture with all its beauty, balance and proportion, and a desire to utilise one's surgical skill, knowledge and experience to create the beauty one has envisaged, then an operating theatre becomes a studio, a surgeon becomes an artist and surgery becomes an art form.
>
> (Alexander, 2007: 166)

As this excerpt suggests, as an aesthetic practice cosmetic surgery is associated with beauty, desire and artistic form and practice.

Constituting the body as an art form, cosmetic surgery opens up into possibilities for 'alternative modes of being and norms' (Gabardi, 2001: 72) relating to the corporeal experience of 'older'. In relation to 'anti-ageing' practices, Cardona (2007: 224) suggests that corporeal enhancement technologies propose 'new standards of normality, success, and moral virtue' that provide 'new benchmarks of what a person should look and act like at a certain age and the desirability of subjecting the body to technoscience and anti-aging treatments in order to alter the "normal" to new values'. The practice of cosmetic surgery within a regimen of self-care thus challenges 'the boundaries of our culture and our selves' (Gabardi, 2001: 127). Furthermore, as Gabardi (2001: 127) elaborates, 'Self-care is an affirmative ethic geared toward the experience of freedom associated with creativity. Conformity is challenged and the self is reflexively refashioned.' From this perspective the notion of 're' introduced at the outset of this chapter in the context of 'anti-ageing' discourse could be reconceived in terms of agency to 're-sculpt' the 'older' body rather than reverse ageing. In Butler's (2004: 107) words, such a practice would 'reinscribe the boundaries of the body along new cultural lines'. Creative self-expression through the aesthetic fashioning of the materiality of the body thus enables new corporeal forms that challenge and exceed the boundaries of 'older' and provide possibilities for looking *better*, rather than 'younger'. However, providing cultural space for these possibilities, as Butler (2001: 20) suggests, 'requires that we break the habits of judgment in favour of a riskier practice that seeks to yield artistry from constraint'.

Summary

The rationality of anti-ageing discourse inscribed in cosmetic surgery practice in relation to 'older' people was problematized in this chapter. Anti-ageing discourse operates to differentiate certain practices of cosmetic surgery as 'anti-ageing' and differentially position 'older' consumers in relation to 'younger' consumers. This is a problem for the cultural politics of 'older' because anti-ageing discourses constitute cosmetic surgery as an ageist practice and 'older' consumers as denying ageing. Such a reductive reading of the body in which age operates to norm appearance, retains a latent essentialism premised upon the constitution of the 'naturally ageing body'. Privileging the discourse articulated by participants that cosmetic surgery is practiced to look *better* not younger, and following Pitts-Taylor (2009: 126), it was suggested that this distinction links the practice of cosmetic surgery to aesthetic concerns that matter because they are 'deeply superficial'. To elaborate the significance of this distinction, alternative rationalities inscribed in cosmetic surgery in relation to a regimen of self-care were explored. Here, cosmetic surgery was situated as a practice of self, discursively positioned at the nexus between technology for aesthetic enhancement (self-improvement), therapeutic intervention (self-fulfilment) and consumer choice (self-indulgence). As a practice of the self, cosmetic surgery can be understood as embedded in the context of neoliberal consumer culture whereby ethical care of self occurs through self-fashioning an appearance and 'lifestyle' in the aestheticization of everyday life. Drawing on Foucault's conceptualization of care of self as an ethic of creativity and freedom, suggests that through aesthetic and creative sensibilities the practice of cosmetic surgery enables possibilities for challenging and exceeding normative limitations concerning how the 'older' body should appear. A question that arises from this discussion, and pursued in what follows, is how cosmetic surgery is engaged to stylize the subjective experience of 'older'.

Notes

1 Parts of this chapter were published as an article: Reprinted from *Journal of Aging Studies*, 27, Garnham, B. (2013) Designing 'Older' rather than Denying Ageing: A Critique of Anti-ageing Discourse in Relation to Cosmetic Surgery Undertaken by Older People, 38–46. with permission from Elsevier.

2 The notion of 'growing old naturally' is taken up and problematized in Chapter 5.
3 Chapter 5 provides discussion of socio-economic status.
4 Despite its long association with psychology, as Heyes (2007) observes, there is little to no evidence of the long term psychological effects or benefits of undergoing cosmetic surgery.

References

Alexander, L. 2007. Fine Art. *Cosmetic Surgery Magazine*. New South Wales: Bella Media.

Bell, D., Holliday, R., Jones, M., Probyn, E. & Taylor, J. S. 2011. Bikinis and Bandages: An Itinerary for Cosmetic Surgery Tourism. *Tourist Studies*, 11, 139–155.

Besley, T. A. C. & Peters, M. A. 2007. *Subjectivity and Truth: Foucault, Education and the Culture of the Self*. New York: Peter Lang Publishing.

Butler, J. 2001. *What is Critique? An Essay on Foucault's Virtue* [Online]. Available: http://www.law.berkeley.edu/centers/kadish/what%20is%20critique%20J%20Butler.pdf [Accessed 30 August 2006].

Butler, J. 2004. Bodily Inscriptions, Performative Subversions. In: Salih, S. & Butler, J. (eds) *The Judith Butler Reader*. USA: Blackwell Publishing.

Cardona, B. 2007. 'Anti-Aging Medicine' and the Cultural Context of Aging in Australia. *Annals of the New York Academy of Sciences*, 1114, 216–229.

Cardona, B. 2008. 'Healthy Ageing' Policies and Anti-ageing Ideologies and Practices: On the Exercise of Responsibility. *Medicine, Health Care and Philosophy*, 11, 475–483.

Cosmetic Surgery Consultants. 2008. *Anti-ageing Surgery* [Online]. Available: http://www.cosmeticsurgeryconsultants.co.uk/anti-aging.htm [Accessed 28 October 2009].

Crawford, R. 1980. Healthism and the Medicalization of Everyday Life. *International Journal of Health Services*, 10, 365–388.

Crawford, R. 2006. Health as a Meaningful Social Practice. *Health: An Interdisciplinary Journal for the Social Study of Health, Illness and Medicine*, 10, 401–420.

Daniels, N. 2002. So What's Wrong With Wrinkles? *The Times*.

DukemedNews. 2005. Older Generation Looking Younger.

Elliot, C. 2003. *Better than Well: American Medicine Meets the American Dream*. New York: W.W Norton & Company.

Featherstone, M. 2007. *Consumer Culture and Postmodernism*. London: Sage Publications.

Fishman, J. R., Binstock, R. H. & Lambrix, M. A. 2008. Anti-aging Science: The Emergence, Maintenance and Enhancement of a Discipline. *Journal of Aging Studies*, 22, 295–303.

Foucault, M. 1990. *The Care of the Self: The History of Sexuality Volume 3*. London: Penguin Books.

Foucault, M. 1994. The Ethic of Care for the Self as a Practice of Freedom. In: Bernauer, J. & Rasmussen, D. (eds) *The Final Foucault*. Cambridge: The MIT Press.

Foucault, M. 2005. *The Hermeneutics of the Subject: Lectures at the College De France 1981–1982*. New York: Picador.

Frank, A. W. 2002. What's Wrong with Medical Consumerism? In: Henderson, S. & Petersen, A. (eds) *Consuming Health*. London: Routledge.

Frank, A. W. & Jones, T. 2003. Bioethics and the Later Foucault. *Journal of Medical Humanities*, 24, 179–186.

FreedoniaGroup. 2005. *Anti-ageing Products to 2009* [Online]. Available: http://www.piribo.com/publications/treatments/antiaging.html [Accessed 28 October 2009].

Gabardi, W. 2001. *Negotiating Postmodernism*. Minneapolis: University of Minnesota Press.

Gilleard, C. & Higgs, P. 2000. *Cultures of Ageing: Self, Citizen and the Body*. Essex: Prentice Hall.

Grove, V. 2000. 'Under The Knife I Find The Real Me'. *The Times*, 26 February.

Haiken, E. 1997. *Venus Envy: A History of Cosmetic Surgery*. Baltimore and London: The John Hopkins University Press.

Hamilton, A. 2006. Not-so-wrinklies Line up for Facelifts. *The Times*, 29 May.

Health Care Complaints Commission. 1999. *The Cosmetic Surgery Report*.

Heyes, C. 2007. *Self-transformations: Foucault, Ethics, and Normalised Bodies*. New York: Oxford University Press.

Higgs, P., Leontowitsch, M., Stevenson, F. & Rees Jones, I. 2009. Not just Old and Sick – The 'Will to Health' in Later Life. *Ageing & Society*, 29, 687–707.

Hilton, L. 2002. Older Americans Have Special Cosmetic Surgery Needs. *Cosmetic Surgery Times Special Reports*, 1 June.

Holliday, R., Bell, D., Cheung, O., Jones, M. & Probyn, E. 2015. Brief Encounters: Assembling Cosmetic Surgery Tourism. *Social Science & Medicine*, 124, 298–304.

Jones, M. 2004. Mutton Cut Up as Lamb: Mothers, Daughters and Cosmetic Surgery. *Continuum: Journal of Media and Cultural Studies*, 18, 525–539.

Linnell, G. 1999. You Beauty. *Bulletin with Newsweek*, 16 November.

Media Monitors. 2007. *Discussion on Various Aspects of Cosmetic Surgery*. Radio. Australia.

Morton, K. 2015. Emerging Geographies of Disciplining the Ageing Body: Practising Cosmetic Technologies in the Aesthetic Clinic. *Gender, Place & Culture*, 22, 1041–1057.

Munro, P. 2009. *Baby Boomers Rage against Age* [Online]. The Age. Available: http://www.theage.com.au/national/baby-boomers-rage-against-age-20090606-bz8g.html [Accessed 28 October 2009].

Murray, S. 2005. (Un/Be)Coming Out? Rethinking Fat Politics. *Social Semiotics*, 15, 153–163.

Mykytyn, C. E. 2006. Anti-aging Medicine: A Patient/Practitioner Movement to Redefine Aging. *Social Science and Medicine*, 62, 643–653.

Nash, M. 2009. Foreign Bodies. *Sunday Life, The Sun-Herald*.

Öberg, P. 2003. Image versus Experience of the Aging Body. In: Faircloth, C. A. (ed.) *Aging Bodies: Images and Everyday Experience*. Walnut Creek: AltMira Press.

Online, M. 2006. *Cosmetic Surgery Helps to Make Sixties New Middle Age* [Online]. Available: www.medicalsearch.com.au/news/printarticle.asp?id=23061 [Accessed 1 June 2007].

Pitts-Taylor, V. 2009. Becoming/Being a Cosmetic Surgery Patient: Semantic Instability and the Intersubjective Self. *Studies in Gender & Sexuality*, 10, 119–128.

Pitts, V. 2006. The Body, Beauty, and Psychosocial Power. In: Chen, N. N. & Moglen, H. (eds) *Bodies in the Making: Transgressions and Transformations*. Santa Cruz: New Pacific Press.

Rose, N. 1996. *Inventing our Selves: Psychology, Power, and Personhood*. Cambridge: Cambridge University Press.

Rose, N. 2001. The Politics of Life Itself. *Theory, Culture & Society*, 18, 1–30.

Rose, N. 2007. *The Politics of Life Itself: Biomedicine, Power, and Subjectivity in the Twenty-First Century*. New Jersey: Princeton University Press.

Ryan, D. 2001. Adding Years Gracefully. *The Age.*

The British Association of Aesthetic Plastic Surgeons. 2005. *Plastic Surgery: It's Not Teens, It's Their Grandparents!* [Online]. London, UK. Available: http://www.baaps.org.uk/content/view/131/62/ [Accessed 13 March 2008].

The Canadian Press. 2002. More People 65 and Older Getting Cosmetic Surgery. 24 July.

World Health Organization. 1948. *Preamble to the Constitution of the World Health Organization* [Online]. New York. Available: http://www.who.int/about/definition/en/print.html [Accessed 13 March 2008].

5 Ageing *dis*gracefully and *becoming* 'older'[1]

Introduction

In *The Use of Pleasure*, Foucault (1990: 10–11) suggests that individuals engage in practices of self in order to 'make their life into an *oeuvre* that carries certain aesthetic values and meets certain stylistic criteria'. In this chapter, aesthetic values and stylistic criteria are explored in relation to a cultural politics of 'older' that informs cosmetic surgery engagement for 'older' people. Firstly, the ethical and aesthetic principles of 'ageing gracefully' and 'mutton dressed as lamb' are problematized in terms of their delimitation of the stylization of 'older' through discourses of 'natural ageing'. The cultural politics suggested by 'ageing naturally' promotes acceptance and display of the 'naturally aged' body. However, the essentialism inherent to such an approach will fail to transform the system that positions these 'aged' bodies as undesirable. Rather, what is needed is a problematization of 'youth' in aesthetics to imagine aesthetically desiring and desirable 'older' bodies. This chapter mobilizes participants' suggestion of a cultural politics of 'ageing *dis*-gracefully' in relation to Foucault's suggestion that ethical self-stylization involves voluntary insubordination to the modes of subjection that attempt to constitute individuals as particular subjects. It explores the stylization of 'older' selves and lifestyles, in terms of contemporary ethico-political discourses, to suggest the reflexive self-fashioning of 'older' can be understood in terms of a 'critical ontology' that elaborates 'older' according to new possibilities and practices.

The ethical principles of 'ageing gracefully' and 'mutton dressed as lamb'

The notion of 'ageing gracefully' operates as an ethical principle that suggests 'older' people should accept 'natural' bodily ageing with a certain aesthetic style and grace. In our interview, when I asked James about the increasing numbers of 'older' people having cosmetic surgery he responded, 'Why they do that I don't know, why they can't be content to grow old gracefully and leave it at that I don't know'. When prompted to define what he meant by growing 'old gracefully' James replied 'Just let things take their course – naturally'. Asked to further elaborate, James stated:

> We've often said, even a situation where people dye their hair when they get older, they've got an old wrinkled face, and dyed hair. It doesn't look right. An old wrinkled face should have grey hair, it's natural. I don't know whether you agree with that, but we have often said that. Even when you get older, you see a man with a big mop of hair; it doesn't always look natural, because old men very often don't have mops of hair. If that is how they are well that is how they are, but we have often said that people who dye their hair shouldn't really do that, because it doesn't look natural.

Given that 'ageing gracefully' is associated with the 'natural' body, surgical intervention to modify the 'older' body is anathema to this notion. In media texts the notion of 'ageing naturally' is often evoked in relation to famous actresses who, it is claimed, have not had cosmetic surgery:

> The non-plastic face French actress Catherine Deneuve, 60, is ageing beautifully in the gentle hands of mother nature.
>
> (Tulloch, 2004)

> Famous beauties who've chosen to age naturally…These three legendary actresses [Lauren Bacall, Brigitte Bardot, Maggie Smith] are, like Dalma, well into their senior years. But instead of altering their appearance as they aged, these symbols of film-star glamour are happy to show their naturally lined faces. As Lauren Bacall insists, 'I have friends who are beautiful women and they're having liposuction and boob lifts and I say, 'What are you doing to yourselves, stop it!' I distain this whole youth-sickness thing.
>
> (Brown, 2006)

These extracts suggest that ageing naturally is associated with beauty and choice. As these examples demonstrate, 'standards of the "natural" are seemingly functioning to establish normative limits of the acceptable' (Weiss and Kukla, 2009: 124).

When I asked James what he would think if someone in their eighties or older had cosmetic surgery he responded:

> I would be disgusted. Very often I have seen women who look like that, honestly I feel physically ill. It makes me feel absolutely horrible. When my partner and I have been out places Festival Theatre or a theatre somewhere and we see an old lady that is painted with dyed hair, she looks absolutely dreadful. On the other hand we've seen elderly ladies who look elegant, nice, no dyed hair, tastefully made up, they look a million dollars, and the difference is so obvious.

That James takes offence to 'older' 'painted' ladies is evident in his physical and verbal expression of disgust. Ahmed (2004) conceptualizes disgust as a corporeal response to 'bad taste'. Whilst Ahmed intends this to mean the sensory act of tasting using the tongue, it might, in this case be applied to an aesthetic sensibility. Through James' expression of disgust, the appearance of these 'painted ladies' is constituted as disgusting. In contrast, James suggests that 'tastefully made up' 'elderly ladies' with 'no dyed hair' are 'elegant' and look 'nice'. I followed up his response by asking what he thought made the difference and he replied 'maybe desperation. I don't know why a lady would want to look like mutton dressed as lamb'. What this statement suggests is that the disgust James feels is anchored by the belief that 'older' women should appear 'age- appropriate' and that the use of cosmetics is an act of desperately trying to style one's appearance like that of a younger person. The notion of 'mutton dressed as lamb' therefore refers to an aesthetic sensibility pertaining to 'older' and operates as an ethical imperative to stylize one's appearance in ways that are considered congruent with one's age.

Together, the ethical principles of 'ageing gracefully' and 'mutton dressed as lamb' suggest that 'older' people should accept 'natural ageing' and stylize an 'age-appropriate' appearance. An inherent paradox resides at the interface of these aesthetic principles whereby graceful acceptance of the 'naturally' ageing body is achieved through its stylization. This paradox, of undertaking body work to 'age naturally', is evident in the contrast James makes between 'painted' ladies and those 'tastefully made up' given that both suggest the use of cosmetic products. When I asked Dr Smith what she thought growing old gracefully means she responded:

> I don't think they know. I think they think that they'd like to look like Sophia Loren when they're seventy not realising that in fact Sophia Loren has had work done… I mean how do you grow old gracefully? … I guess, you know, they'd like to be beautiful and serene and grow old. I mean that's not exactly the real world is it?

Dr Smith suggests that those people who aspire to 'ageing gracefully' and being 'beautiful and serene' don't realize Sophia Loren has had 'work done'.[2] I read her assertion 'I mean that's not exactly the real world is it?' to suggest that 'ageing gracefully' entails body work rather than passive acceptance of 'natural' ageing.

Ms Robinson explicitly associates 'ageing gracefully' with active engagement in practices to take care of the body:

> the only ones who, I believe, really take care of their skin are the ones who have had a problem when they are young like acne or, you know, eczema or…You know they're the ones who tend to age a lot more gracefully, I think because they haven't taken their skin for granted.

Similarly, Ms Taylor and Dr Wilson both suggest that 'older' people who 'look good' have been able to engage in practices to 'take care of themselves':

> I look at my parents now and they don't look anything like sixty-five year olds. But occasionally you still see one that comes in and it's quite, yeah, a bit taken aback, you think "God they're only sixty-five. That's really young. Why do they look so bad?" But socio-economic has a lot to do with it I think. The less money you have, the less time you spend keeping yourself looking good.
>
> (Ms Taylor)

> I mean a lot of these people in their fifties, sixties, you know, sixties, seventies, you look at them, have a look, just have a look at people generally. I mean not so much the ones in the old folks home who are frail and things like that, you know, but sometimes you look at them, you know, people are all fit and healthy at the beach, they care of themselves and things like that… And why [do they look good]? A lot of these people they spent a lot of time taking care of themselves when they were younger and, you look at them, even now, they still look very good for their age, very fit for their age. So just to take care of themselves. I mean because it's when you let go, that's when you know, it just goes.
>
> (Dr Wilson)

The aesthetic style and grace associated with 'ageing gracefully' may therefore entail taking care of the self through practices that cultivate the body rather than passive acceptance of 'natural' bodily ageing (also see Chapter 4).

Foucault's analyses of the inscription of power in the materiality of the body suggest that the 'natural' body is a discursive production anchored in biological 'truth' that informs the normative body. Given this theorization of the body, the 'path to aging "naturally" is highly problematic' since 'If there is no natural body, then there is no natural way to age' (Twigg, 2004: 63). If there is no 'natural' body then the notion of 'ageing gracefully' can be reconfigured to represent the pinnacle of a lifelong regimen of 'taking care of oneself'. The metaphor evoked by 68 year old Atthalin captures this point. She states, 'I've been involved with my body and healing and my health for 40 years…It's like I'm a tree. I've been growing for 68 years and now I am going to enjoy the fruit' (Kornblum, 2004). Cosmetic surgery as a practice of self-care however, is not without its attendant risks.

Risky practices and plastic selves: passing as natural

What is the difference between having cosmetic surgery and engaging in aesthetic practices deemed 'acceptable' under the rubric of 'ageing gracefully'? One media extract states 'Creams, cosmetics and hair colour are one thing: procedures that involve anaesthetics, scalpels and needles are another' (Daniels,

2002). This media article differentially positions medical and surgical practices against 'everyday' practices such as the use of cosmetics and hair colour. The problematization that underpins this distinction is the constitution of cosmetic surgery as invasive, extreme and risky compared to non-invasive, conservative and relatively safe cosmetic practices. Chloe states:

> cosmetic surgery is really about how far you would go, yes. Really cosmetic surgery is the end of the line. I think you would do a lot of things before you get to that point to spend many thousands of dollars and take a risk.

This statement constitutes the difference between cosmetic surgery and other aesthetic practices in terms of degree rather than substance.

The risks associated with cosmetic surgery are not only medical risks associated with having a surgical procedure but also social and aesthetic. The social risks, as previously described, entail judgement for trying to deny 'natural' ageing and thus the risk of being stigmatized. As Elliot (2003: 108) has observed 'The stigma is rooted in worries about fakery and passing, of trying to hide the person you really are'. In terms of avoiding stigma it is therefore important that the post-surgical body is read as 'natural'.

The discursive influence of the 'natural' body was evident in statements concerning the desired appearance of the post-surgical modified body. Fears of appearing 'plastic' or residual evidence of surgical intervention and thus being unable to 'pass' as natural were the outworking of this powerful influence:

> This is the most successful response to surgery – simply to look well and happier. 'It would be a failure,' says Waterhouse, 'if you walked into a room and people said, 'Hey, you've had your face done.' 'People want to look rested and fresh-faced. They don't want that tight-pulled Nancy Reagan-Joan Rivers look (like a Siamese cat walking into the teeth of a gale, as Lynda Smith, the comedienne, says), but just a better version of themselves.
>
> (Grove, 2000)

> It looks so natural, people don't notice.
>
> (Grove, 2000)

> Today's cosmetic surgery was designed to follow the natural structure of a face, and should not result in the wide-eyed, stretched look of yesteryear.
>
> (Robotham, 2004)

As these excerpts suggest, the pressure is on surgeons to conceal any evidence of surgery. Dr Brown acknowledges this ambition when he states:

> So if you do an operation, cosmetic procedure and there's no trails, then we are very happy and have a celebratory red wine at night. We've done,

> very, very good work, it's healed beautifully, the patient's achieved the outcome, and there's no signs. That's the ultimate.

Similarly, Dr Cooper explained that he aims for an outcome whereby the patient 'will look like they have not been operated on. That is, that it could have been the way they were born.' I asked many of the surgeons interviewed what they would do if a patient asked for an appearance that fell beyond the boundaries of what they considered 'normal', 'natural' or achievable and all emphatically insisted that they would refuse the surgery or 'recalibrate' the patient's expectations.

In terms of 'older', the risk of being unable to pass as natural following cosmetic surgery was posed in relation to bodily incongruence. In the texts generated for this book, Heather articulates this risk best in her narrative that she was walking down the street when

> this beautiful face came towards me with the lipstick perfectly on, the perfect mouth and the eyes. It was a glorious face…But it was the old body. And I kept thinking to myself that woman is beautiful but what's wrong with her? She had a young face on a very old body. So I think that you have to get plastic surgery everywhere when you get the face done.

Ms Harris speaks to the same notion of bodily incongruence when she states 'if they've still got a lot of skin pigmentations and that then their skin will be tighter but the skin quality won't be as [good], it will still be aged'. This excerpt suggests that skin pigmentation would 'give away' the 'aged body' despite tighter skin.

Another risk of having cosmetic surgery was that of 'age-inappropriateness'. For example, I asked Ms Robinson what she would think of a 70 or 75 year old who had undergone breast augmentation and she replied, 'disgusting… Because their skin is not even the same, the elasticity is not there. They look aged but they've got these full looking breasts, it doesn't look natural.' Interestingly, Charlotte told me that whilst she would love to have some botox injected into some lines she had decided not to because those lines were probably helping her 'get away with taking away the other lines'. Being able to 'get away with' having cosmetic surgery suggests being able to 'pass' as natural and maintain bodily congruence and age-appropriateness.

Given that cosmetic surgery constitutes a technological intervention undertaken to transform the body and self, the discursive construction of the 'natural' body limits corporeal-stylization and makes cosmetic surgery a risky practice. As Weiss and Kukla (2009: 117) assert, the 'natural look' in cosmetic surgery discourse entails an 'essentialist position that imposes ethical limits on those transformations in the name of nature'. As they elaborate, this entails a 'complex message that normative, "natural" bodies can be the product of artifice and technology' (Weiss & Kukla, 2009: 121). In terms of aesthetic sensibilities, 'natural' is therefore deployed to set norms that constitute and limit corporeal transformations. The essentialism of this discourse reinforces the apparatus that constitutes 'older' in terms of normative 'natural' bodies. However, these norms are not fixed and so the practice of cosmetic surgery may still work to unsettle, transgress and reinscribe norms that govern the appearance of 'older' bodies.

The cultural politics of ageing gracefully

Given the suggestion that 'celebrities who choose to age naturally' are taking a 'laudable' stand (Daniels, 2002), 'ageing gracefully' entails a political dimension. According to this media article, celebrities are taking a stand against cosmetic surgery and the 'ideal of youth' that drives the consumption of products to 'deny ageing'. Being 'daring' enough and 'happy' to show natural lines and wrinkles is thus considered a political statement that challenges 'youthful' aesthetic ideals (Daniels, 2002). The article concludes that 'The power to change attitudes is in our hands'. 'Ageing naturally' is therefore positioned as an act of resistance that will alter attitudes concerning the 'aged body'. Such a position extols the ethical virtues of the 'natural' body and suggests that this body is less constrained by relations of power. In the academic literature, Hurd Clarke and Griffin (2007: 189) are among those who suggest 'the natural body that has not submitted to ageist and patriarchial definitions of beauty and femininity and corresponding body work interventions is superior or, at the very least, less constrained by ageism and sexist oppression'. A parallel can be drawn here between the politics associated with 'ageing naturally' and 'fat politics'. As Murray (2005: 161) suggests, the 'fat body' like the 'aged body', 'is positioned outside of dominant aesthetic ideals'. Drawing on Sedgwick's work, Murray describes the notion inherent to 'fat politics' that you must 'speak' your fatness and 'come out' as fat. She elaborates that this is a 'central tenet of the philosophy of most size acceptance organisations; that is, that we should learn to love our fat bodies, and make them visible in new, enabling, and politically empowering ways' (Murray, 2005: 160). Political statements of 'ageing naturally' promote a similar acceptance and display of the 'aged body' to challenge aesthetic values.

Murray (2005: 162), however, questions the efficacy of 'the simple reversal from a negative body to a celebrated one'. Such an approach is limited, she argues, because 'the system of judgement that positions the fat body as a negative body *remains intact*' (Murray, 2005: 162 emphasis in original). Murray quotes Sullivan's text (Sullivan, 2003 cited in Murray, 2005: 153) on queer politics to argue that 'The call to come out presupposes that such an action is in itself transformative and that the identity that one publically declares is unambiguous'. Similarly, Probyn (2008: 402) has pointed out that 'The idea that politics can be served by methodologically simply effecting a semiotic reversal has been deeply critiqued by many'. She argues that in this approach to 'fat politics', 'fat becomes objectified as a mode of resistance' and subjectivity is reduced to 'fat woman' (Probyn, 2008: 402). 'As a viable strategy for social intervention' she suggests, 'this is painfully limited, and can have quite disastrous political consequences' (Probyn, 2008: 403). She also laments that this is 'a sad way to understand human subjectivity' (Probyn, 2008: 403). The insights offered by Murray, Sullivan and Probyn suggest that objectifying the 'aged body' as a mode of resistance and reducing 'older' to corporeal signification is limited in terms of its potential to transform the relations of power that constitute normative bodies as 'youthful'.

Probyn (2008) suggests that much of the work that supports this limited notion of 'fat politics' is based on a narrow reading of Foucault's work on disciplinary power and resistance. According to this reading, bodies are disciplined and subjected as 'docile' in relation to a system of norms by practices such as dieting, cosmetic surgery, gym regimens. Refusing to engage in these techniques and practices is thus read as a mode of resistance. However, as Foucault's later work on ethical practices of self suggests, and Chapter 1 and Chapter 4 have argued, these techniques can also be read as practices of self-care that constitute the ethical subject. The problem inherent to these politics is, as Murray (2005: 159, emphasis in original) asks, 'How can you completely remove yourself from the discourses that *constitute us as subjects*?'

The significance of this question resides in Foucault's conceptualization of discourse as practices that have effects in the real. Practices of self have the power to shape our subjective experience in terms such as self-esteem, confidence, happiness, and overall self-fulfilment and wellbeing (see Chapter 4). Murray for example, confesses her own desire to be thin as a desire to experience being aesthetically and sexually desirable. She argues that this demonstrates that 'fat acceptance' remains an ambivalent position with respect to normative bodies. By sustaining a system of mutually exclusive dichotomies that intersect with desirable/undesirable, such as thin/fat, youthful/aged, young/old, along with Murray (2005: 162), I suggest that these politics refuse 'the possibilities ambiguity presents'. What is needed is a reading that breaks down these dichotomies to consider the practice of cosmetic surgery by 'older' people outside 'youthful ideals'. Such a reading works to problematize 'youth' in aesthetics and imagine aesthetically desiring and desirable 'older' bodies.

Problematizing 'youth' in aesthetics: desiring and desirable 'older' bodies

Drawing on Bourdieu's notion of 'habitus', Tulle (2008: 7) argues that we can 'conceive of age itself as a structure guiding our social location and our dispositions'. In terms of aesthetic sensibilities and dispositions, age structures what is considered desirable and appropriate according to one's social location in the life-course. The ethical and stylistic principles of 'ageing naturally' and 'mutton dressed as lamb' emerge from this 'habitus'. Age however, also becomes enmeshed in aesthetics through notions such as 'youthful' aesthetic ideals, consumer culture as 'youth culture' and society as obsessed with 'youth'. That these notions have become culturally taken for granted is apparent in their treatment as self-evident in many of the texts and literature generated for this book. Through this entanglement, 'old is opposed to young and any quality associated with youth cannot be attributed to the old' (Tulle, 2008: 3). Such a rendering excludes the possibility of desirable and desiring 'older' bodies.

Prefigured by notions of 'youth' in aesthetics, scholarship on ageing and the body has raised concerns regarding the social and cultural marginalization of the 'aged body' (see for example, Hepworth, 2003; Powell and Longino, 2001; Shilling, 2003; Turner, 1995; Twigg, 2004). Powell and Longino (2001: 204) for example, assert that 'Consumer culture marginalizes the identity of older people by emphasizing youthfulness, the "body beautiful"'. Similarly, Twigg (2004: 61) argues that:

> Consumer culture is quintessentially youth culture in that it presents and promotes youthfulness as the ideal; and this has profound consequences for how we experience aging in high- or postmodernity. The bodies featured in the media are never old; and the emphasis on perfectionism and the visible eradication of age is reinforced in the growing industry of age denial.

According to this perspective, in the aestheticization of everyday life, the 'aged body' is constituted as a disruption of the visual field (Furman, 1999 cited in Twigg, 2004) and largely rendered socially and culturally invisible. In a study concerning the 'aged body' and the media, Vares (2009) explores depictions of the 'Sexy Oldie' in film. She argues that some participants' affective responses of disgust to a filmic image of a naked, sexually active woman in her sixties, work to constitute it as 'unwatchable' (Vares, 2009: 503). 'Youthful' aesthetic ideals thus constitute the visible, desirable and desiring body as young bodies. The effect of this, Gilleard and Higgs (2000: 62), suggest, is that the only culturally sanctioned action within a '"staying young" culture' is to engage in 'anti-ageing' technologies to deny and resist ageing.

Given that the 'body beautiful' constitutes an aesthetic *ideal*, it seems unlikely that 'older' people experience these ideals any differently to any other age group since bodies of all ages are marginalized by such ideals in multi-layered ways. Moreover, 'youthful' aesthetic ideals suggest that younger bodies are universally desirable. Whilst it would seem apparent that this is hardly the case, this notion has become a taken-for-granted assumption in much of the writing around aesthetics and aesthetic practices. A question that captivates the imaginary in this chapter is whether the 'body beautiful', generally constituted as toned, slender, fit and smooth, has to necessarily be young?

Tulle-Winton (2000) showed undergraduate student nurses photos of journalist and actress Nettie Harris whilst in her late seventies and early eighties and in which she was nude or semi-nude.[3] Tulle-Winton (2000: 71) writes:

> The student nurses declared the photographs almost acceptable because she had a slim body – a good figure for her age, as they put it – thus

> making them just about worth showing. But most of the time they found the photographs disturbing because they showed the body of an old woman in unconventional and ambiguous ways.

This statement suggests that whilst the students' aesthetic sensibilities concerning the visual body were confronted and challenged by 'unconventional and ambiguous' images, they found the photographs 'almost acceptable' due to the slenderness of the depicted body.

Similarly, in a study concerning the visual portrayal of the sexually active older person in film, Bildtgård (2000: 174) suggests that the condition of acceptance for the desiring and desirable 'older' body is that 'the body must be "well preserved", meaning that it is aesthetic and functional'. What these insights seem to suggest is that 'age' might be suspended in aesthetic judgements if the form of corporeal flesh meets certain stylistic criteria. Whilst it is hardly insightful to suggest that the visual body needs to meet certain stylistic criteria to be considered aesthetically desirable, the notion that 'youth' can be detached from aesthetic judgement suggests that 'older' can be associated with its own aesthetic sensibilities.

'Ageing celebrities' are often championed or criticized in relation to whether they are 'ageing well'. Amongst those celebrities featured in the media texts in this study Helen Mirren, Judi Dench, Meryl Streep, Maggie Smith and Joan Bakewell were among those 'older' women whose beauty is celebrated. An article on the cosmetic surgery website MakeMeHeal.com (2007) uses the 2007 nomination of Helen Mirren, Judi Dench and Meryl Streep for an Academy Award for Best Actress as an imprimatur to comment on whether or not these actresses appear to have undergone any cosmetic surgery. Whilst the article suggests that all three may have undergone particular cosmetic procedures, it is the proclamation that these actresses 'exude sexiness, elegance and class' and are 'poised to redefine beauty' that drew my attention. The conclusion to the article states:

> With one of these ladies set to win the Oscar, it will be a triumph for beauty at any age. We congratulate Helen Mirren, Meryl Streep, and Judi Dench for being towering acting talents with beauty to match and appreciate their role in setting new beauty standards for our society.

An article such as this may be read as a marketing strategy to promote particular cosmetic surgery procedures. However, the mode through which such advertising becomes successful is through the promotion of the desirable in order to generate desire.

The following media extract refers to television presenter Anne Robinson to suggest that the surgically enhanced 'older' body can be desirable and generate desire:

> Stunning examples like Robinson's probably explain why a growing number of men and women over the age of sixty are opting to go under a plastic surgeon's knife.
>
> (Alphamaleblog, 2006)

As an aesthetic and creative practice (See Chapter 4) cosmetic surgery has the potential[4] to generate desire for corporeal enhancement and optimization, and create desirable corporal forms that 'in turn construct more desire/pleasure' (Besley and Peters, 2007: 45).

Aesthetically desirable images of the 'older' body in the media operate as ideals. These ideals and those that fashion themselves in relation to these ideals challenge presumptions about how the 'older' body should and could appear. That normative expectations regarding an 'older' appearance have and are continuing to be modified is evident in Ms Taylor's observations that 'most of my parent's generation are mid sixties and they don't look anything like a sixty year old did when I was a kid'. Interestingly, it is through media depiction of the desirable 'older' body that the visibility of 'older' people in the media is being increased. This has the potential to challenge the universalizing of 'youthful' ideals, 'youth culture' and a society obsessed with 'youth'. In light of this, to continue to refer to consumer culture as 'youth culture' would be to perpetuate the boundaries that constrain 'older' and work to exclude and marginalize 'older' people. When I asked Dr Smith how she thought society at large views older people wanting to have cosmetic surgery she replied 'disgusting'. When asked to elaborate she replied, 'because we're hypocrites. And because fun and life and alcohol and sex and beauty and drugs are all only for young people. And I think it's an extension of that'. I asked whether she was suggesting that this was a form of ageism and she stated:

> Absolutely. 'Why do they bother?' I think younger people view it like that. A lot of their peers would probably…I mean some people think, you know, 'Good on you, wish I could do it, don't have the courage, the money' the whatever. Some people would think that it's silly. I think the general opinion would be 'Ick'. 'Why do they bother, they're old anyway.'

As Dr Smith suggests, it is not necessarily consumer culture that is ageist but rather the exclusion of 'older' people from engaging in consumer culture and practices. Similarly, it is not cosmetic surgery practice that is necessarily ageist but cultural tropes such as 'graceful ageing' when this is taken to mean that 'older' people should be proud of their 'naturally' aged bodies and those who continue to engage in practices of self-care are shamed and denigrated.

In ageing studies scholarship much has been made of the cultural changes being driven by the large cohort now entering older ages referred to as the 'baby boomers'. The generation of the post-Second World War baby boom, the baby boomers were the 'youth' that drove the development of 'youth culture' in the 'cultural revolution of the 1960s' (Gilleard and Higgs, 2002: 378).

Credited with challenging and transforming culture throughout the lifecourse, the babyboomers and 'ageing' of post war youth culture are now 'confounding ideas of what it means to be "old"' (Gilleard and Higgs, 2000: 9). As with the development of 'youth culture' before it, the development and transformation of cultures of 'older' will be driven through and represented within consumer culture and practices. In terms of appearance and consumerism, Chris suggests that:

> Just because people are older doesn't mean that they don't want to appear good in front of their peers. Older people get portrayed a bit too often as frumpy, lumpy and dumb and get ignored by major marketing chains, by market advertising campaigns. If you are over 28 forget it you are old, go away. Older people are too often regarded that way. But I don't think they think that way.

The baby boomers are a significant cohort of consumers; one that is increasingly being recognized and targeted as a potential market in advertising campaigns. Such campaigns will need to represent 'older' in terms of new aesthetic sensibilities and practices – to market desirable 'older' bodies and identities and thus generate desire for consumption. Cultural change will therefore be an outworking of this marketization.

The cultural politics of ageing *dis*gracefully

In texts generated for this book, the mechanisms of subjection suggested by 'ageing gracefully' and the stylization of an 'elderly' identity were resisted through a politics of 'ageing *dis*gracefully'. One media text (Ryan, 2001) suggests 'ageing gracefully' is a staid and perhaps outdated notion stating that 'instead of ageing gracefully, the fiftysomethings of today seem intent on ageing outrageously. They are determined to be more active, healthier and have more fun than their predecessors'. When I asked Dr Smith about the notion of ageing gracefully she responded 'not being a particularly graceful person myself I can't imagine ever growing old gracefully. I personally would like to grow old disgracefully'. Similarly, a media article (Potera, 2000) featuring Joan Kron, a 64 year old cosmetic surgery reporter and patient, states, 'If people ask her why she looks younger, better or different, she isn't coy, like many Hollywood stars. She's straightforward and honest, telling those people who ask that she had a facelift. "I call it growing old disgracefully", Kron says'.

Despite the ethical imperative to dress in ways that are considered appropriate for one's age and the risk of being labelled 'mutton dressed as lamb', transgression of 'age-appropriate' norms is deliberate for Sophie and admired by Charlotte. Sophie asserts that she likes to 'dress younger than I am'. She tells me:

> I wear sexy underwear I always have…Somedays I worry when I put my little thongs on the clothes line and then I think oh what the hell with it. People don't like it, their not wearing them, I am.

Similarly, Charlotte comments that:

> My friends are all old, I have a lovely lady who is coming away with me and she is over 90 and I admire her so much. She wears thongs, I can't wear thongs, age is irrelevant to her it really is.

As these statements demonstrate, wearing 'sexy underwear' that transgresses 'age- appropriate' norms is not about trying to appear 'younger' but rather the 'irrelevance of age'.

Charlotte, Mandy and Angela also express this critical attitude in terms of the rhetorical
question 'why not?' when asked about their decisions to have cosmetic surgery:

> Why not? I think it is an attitude also. Why not?
>
> (Charlotte)

> You start off by doing it because you look in the mirror and you might be seeing something that could be tighter and you think why not do it?
>
> (Mandy)

> If you can afford cosmetic surgery, then why not?
>
> (Angela)

In the following excerpts featuring Dalma Edwards, 'Australia's cosmetic surgery queen' (Norris, 2003), the juxtaposition of an 'elderly' identity and age 'inappropriate' behaviour befitting the notion of 'ageing disgracefully' is evident:

> While other people her age were getting hip replacements, Dalma was back under the laser having puffy eyes zapped and rouge wrinkles banished. With her saggy "chook" neck and jowls melted away, Dalma turned 80 with newly plumped lips.
>
> (Norris, 2003)

> "A lot of the old dears don't like me, which can be hurtful", she confides, hospitably offering tea and biscuits. "They're all grey-haired and miserable. They look me up and down and I hear them whispering, It's awful. Why doesn't she act her age? But why should I?"
>
> (Brown, 2006)

These excerpts indicate that Dalma's age group peers are 'getting hip replacements' and are 'grey-haired and miserable' whilst Dalama refuses to 'act her age'. Dalma exclaims, 'Yes, I am a freak,'…'I know that…but I am a happy freak!' (Brown, 2006).

In his work conceptualizing critique as an ethical practice, Foucault (1997: 32) considers the art of voluntary insubordination a virtue. It is this art of voluntary insubordination that ensures the desubjugation of the subject in a 'politics of truth' (Foucault, 1997: 32). For Foucault (1997: 28) this entails a 'critical attitude' and 'an act of defiance' in relation to mechanisms of subjection that operate to render individuals intelligible and govern their conduct. Dalma's question 'why should I?' is an act of defiance that simply and beautifully captures and exemplifies what I believe Foucault meant by voluntary insubordination. Refusing to be constituted as an 'old dear', Dalma's proclamation that she is a 'freak' suggests a position of desubjugation.

The cultural politics of 'ageing disgracefully' is a politics of exceeding the boundaries and limitations that seek to constrain the aesthetic stylization of 'older'. Through the practice of cosmetic surgery 'older' is subject to critique. This, I suggest speaks to a 'politics of possibility' that works through critique to cleave open new spaces in which 'older' might be reflexively self-fashioned. Having engaged and problematized the ethical and stylistic principles associated with the cultural politics of 'older', I now want to address, in depth and at face value, the central contention that 'older' people want to look better, not younger (see Chapter 4) and further explore how people aged 65–75 stylize their embodied experience of 'older'.

Aesthetic stylization of the 'older' self

The suggestion that 'older' is constituted through aesthetic stylization particularly emerged in my interviews with participants in the context of clothing style.[5] Angela referred to the undesirability of dressing 'too young' in her statement that 'obviously you can't go like mutton dressed as lamb with little tights and little skimpy tops. That would be ridiculous wouldn't it?' However, others talked about the undesirability of dressing 'too old'. Emily, for instance, says 'I've got a friend who's 72 and she dresses older than what I do. She dresses like a grandmother'. When I asked her what she meant by this she responded:

> Well nothing modern. Old fashioned. Like she'll look down on some of the things I wear because I like wearing nice casual clothes. What I think is nice anyway. Whereas, I mean in my day the older people wore everything that was dark. No colour. They were really drab and that's sort of how she is. And I don't want to be like that.

Here Emily suggests that dressing 'old' is to wear old fashioned, dark, drab clothing as opposed to the nice casual modern clothes that she chooses for herself. Mandy specifically relates the cosmetic procedures she underwent, including tummy tuck, liposuction and breast reduction, to clothing choice. She states:

> I wasn't wanting to turn the clock back to look 18 again. I just wanted to feel more comfortable in myself with clothes because when you are bigger it's really hard to buy clothes – modern clothes – you know they are all a bit frumpy.

Similarly, Chris suggests that

> Older people who end up with stomachs and fat bums and stuff like that, they don't like the way they look, so in that way they'd like to trim down so they can fit better clothes.

Moreover, Chris explicitly links 'old' with clothing when he states 'Once you get above that [a size 14], you go from stylish clothing to old persons' clothing. By that I mean the stretch jeans'. As this data illustrates, 'old' is constituted through aesthetic stylization in ways that are considered 'drab', 'frumpy' and generally 'unstylish'.

As Gilleard and Higgs (2000: 143) assert, 'people do not want to look old and unattractive'. However, this is more than just an aesthetic preference. When I asked Heather why she thought people in their sixties and seventies were deciding to have cosmetic surgery she responded:

> Oh because, really you don't want me to tell you that do you? I tell you why. Because, you now become, when you get to my age, an invisible person. Look I'm lucky; I know that I'm still not ugly. But I know that a lot of older women are just bypassed and I have seen it and I notice it.

She went on to talk about customer service in shops and a social experiment conducted by the BBC where they:

> dressed a young women as an old woman and got her to go into a shop there was no attention paid to her, she didn't get the service, the guy didn't smile at her. But when she took off all that old garbage and she went back into the shop, the guy, you know she was showing a bit of cleavage and walked in, and the guy was over her to help her.

She concluded that 'if your not fuckable – desirable – then they're not even going to talk to you so that's why'. For Heather personally, appearance is important because she states, 'I still want to be taken seriously as a person so I do not want to look old and drab. What I said to you before about being overlooked as an older person'. More than aesthetics, an 'old and drab' appearance works to socially and culturally position individuals as 'elderly':

> 'Women want to be noticed and not seen as frail old ladies,' he said. 'It's the same kind of thing for men.'
>
> (The Canadian Press, 2002)

> Well people are accepting that I don't look old. No-one treats me old. I am talking about people who are sometimes 40 years younger than me. I am not treated as an old person. My husband is, people leap up and offer him a seat and it makes him so mad.
>
> (Charlotte)

> People treat them differently. I think people treat them like they're perhaps going a bit senile.
>
> (Dr Smith)

> So if they act younger, look younger then they'll treat them in one way and if they act really old and look really old then they'll be more helpful…
>
> (Ms Taylor)

An old and unattractive appearance is therefore not only aesthetically displeasing but entails undesirable social and cultural differentiation in terms of an 'elderly identity'. This speaks to 'a relational self where intersubjectivity becomes central – a self that acknowledges and is constituted by difference and the Other' (Besley and Peters, 2007: 20).

Dr Wilson captures this notion and suggests that being positioned as 'Other', in this case 'elderly', is like being in the 'wrong costume' when he states:

> you know it's like Shakespeare says that, you know, 'We are all actors on a stage'. Well it's the same thing, you see. It's like, you know, it's like what mask you have on your face, you know and you play that role and when you suddenly can't play that role convincingly, how would you feel? It's like you're going on stage to play Hamlet but you look like somebody else, you're in the wrong costume and you have to play that. It's not going to be right is it?

Many of the participants aged 65–75 years that I interviewed for this book explicitly positioned themselves as 'not old'. However, this has less to do with denying or resisting chronological age or 'elderly' as an essential nature than a desire to exceed the boundaries that seek to constrain them, regulate their conduct and determine the nature of their interpersonal relations. As Gilleard and Higgs (2000) assert, 'older' people are happy to age but not be aged. The stylization of 'older' using practices to fashion the appearance of the body is therefore deployed in struggles around subjectivity to challenge, resist and subvert forms of subjectivity connected to being 'aged' or 'elderly'.

Stylization of an active 'older' self and lifestyle

The introduction to this book presented the notion that through the commodification of practices of self, consumer culture provides 'sites of distinction' (Gilleard and Higgs, 2000: 8) for a multiplicity of cultural positions in relation to the experience of 'older'. Amid this growing cultural abundance 'older' individuals reflexively fashion lifestyles. By far the most commonly used adjective in the texts generated for this study to describe 'older' in terms of self and lifestyle was 'active'. Almost all of the 65–75 year old participants in this study described themselves and their lives as 'active'. For Tom being active means 'There is nothing I can't do. I still go ice-skating with the grandkids. I do indoor bowls two nights a week. I dance to every bit of music, I am a crazy dancer. I love dancing.' Tom, Isabella and Mandy, consider an active lifestyle to be a life where you 'make the most out of it'.

Cosmetic surgery to enhance appearance was associated with an active lifestyle comprising, employment, leisure pursuits, socializing and relationships:

> Dr Lawrence R LeWinn, says that patients 65 and older make up 65 percent of his practice. 'They are amazingly active,' he said. 'Many of them insist on surgery in the summer months because it's too hot to play golf here'.
>
> (Stock, 1996)

> People in their middle 60s and 70s are feeling better about themselves. They're still out there working, socially active, and they're concerned about projecting the right image.
>
> (Stock, 1996)

> People are now working into their 60s and 70s and are staying active and therefore continue to take care of the way they look.
>
> (PanipatOnline.com, 2005)

> After Hazel York's husband died, she moved into a retirement home, convinced the better part of her life was over. Then she met Damon. She's 81. He's 78. They were married about a year and a half ago...She feels she won a second chance at life, so she decided to give her face a second chance too...She says she did it [facelift] for herself. 'Don't get me wrong. I don't want to look 16 again,' she said, 'but I also don't want to look like Damon's mother.
>
> (The Canadian Press, 2002)

> Health-conscious 65-year-olds 'realize that they have another 20 to 30 years to socialize' says Brian Kinney, MD, an assistant clinical professor of plastic surgery.
>
> (Potera, 2000)

Rather than desperately trying to 'stay young' and deny ageing, these extracts suggest that stylizing a desirable 'older' appearance is part of an 'active' lifestyle.

One media article (PanipatOnline.com, 2005) cites Douglas McGeorge, president of the British Association of Aesthetic Plastic Surgery as stating, 'We live in a well-off society where people now retire to start a new life'. In our interviews Charlotte and Chloe both suggested that an active 'older' lifestyle is linked to cosmetic surgery and wealth.

> People in their 60s if they decide to have facelifts, they want to and they don't see their age, they see it as an improvement for their time in life and they still have plenty of things they're planning to do – they are going to travel and just live a life. It's not old in their eyes. You have got to get to that age to realize that it is much more fun, life is so much better as you get older, because you own your possessions; you have a choice of whether you want to get more or not.
>
> (Charlotte)

> Well we are fortunate, that 60 and 70 year olds have got to that age feeling good, still living good lifestyles, busy lifestyles, still earning money, able to take trips overseas. Most of us our children have left home and are standing on their own feet, therefore we are financially quite independent and we don't hesitate to spend money and enjoy the years that we have. I think we have quite high expectations, we are not ready to sit in the rocking chair on the veranda by any means, we have things to do and places to go, but we want to look good and if finances are there, yes cosmetic surgery is part of it.
>
> (Chloe)

As these extracts demonstrate, Charlotte and Chloe see 'older' as a time of freedom from financial struggle and being able to enjoy the consumption of commodities. Chris also reflects that money is an important factor in active lifestyles and suggests that such lifestyles may not be available to 'pensioners' relying on social retirement schemes for income.

> Yes it is where your head is in your life. It often comes back to money, where you live, how you live, if you can afford to go out and have a meal, can you afford to go out and go to the cinema, and can you have nice things around you. That all comes back to money, whereas there are a lot of people who are pensioners which is not a very good income, you can't do anything. So they end up being stuck in front of the telly, sitting at home and they almost can't afford to go down the street and have a cup of coffee with a friend. We have a few friends like that who are really stuck in their life and because they are stuck in their life, their whole psyche and their whole way of looking at life just deteriorates down and down and they don't come up again. They lose a spark about being enthusiastic about things.

Clearly, being wealthy enough to be able to afford cosmetic surgery and leisure pursuits such as travel is an individual and social condition for the fashioning of active 'older' lifestyles. As a feature of 'cultures of ageing', fashioning an active lifestyle and self-image is therefore conditioned by economic conditions. Whilst a certain amount of disposable income is needed to engage in the practice of cosmetic surgery and fashion active lifestyles, the 'older' participants interviewed for this book came from a range of socio-economic positions. Whilst Mandy told me that money was not a consideration in her decision to have cosmetic surgery, Isabella spoke of her careful saving plan whereby she put aside small sums until she had saved enough for her procedure.

This 'cultural habitat' (Gill, 2008), comprising employment, wealth, leisure activities, health, social and romantic relationships, is associated with the 'young old' or 'third age' subject. (See, for example, Featherstone, 1995; Gilleard and Higgs, 2000; Gilleard and Higgs, 2013; Katz, 2005; Katz and Laliberte-Rudman, 2005; Katz and Marshall, 2003; Powell, 2006.) Historically and culturally, this demographic category is considered the 'new old' (PanipatOnline.com, 2005). James specifically connects being 'active' with the 'young old' in his statement:

> You can hardly classify yourself as young [old] if you weren't active, could you? If you were 65–75 and you weren't active and you just sat around watching television and reading the newspaper and couldn't go out and do the garden or couldn't do jobs around the house you could hardly be classed as young/old could you? If you weren't able to do things, you wouldn't feel young. If you couldn't do things. I feel as if I am alright because I can still do things. I'm active.

In the following statement Chloe suggests the importance of lifestyle to the new cultural constitution of the 'young old'.

> I don't think today's 70 year old is anything like the last 20 years ago or my parent's age. Sadly my mother didn't live beyond 62 but I think I am probably a younger 70 year old than she would have been and I think the next generation will be extremely young at 70 because we are lucky we can maintain a healthy, fit lifestyle. As long as you don't get any dreaded disease or health problems, no reason we shouldn't go on for many more years. It is the maintenance! – the vitamins, the good food and I think mental health is important. Your mental attitude to everything is important.

As this extract suggests, maintaining a 'healthy, fit lifestyle' and 'mental attitude' is a condition of possibility for the constitution of the 'active' 'young old'. Chloe links being 'active' with physical and mental health in her statement that:

> I think because there are a lot of us now who are active, you look into the political world, the arts world, the music world, the business world.

> There are plenty of 60–65, 70 year olds still doing a great job with a lot to offer. These days I don't think the older generation hits 60 and thinks I must retire now, they are happy to keep working for various reasons but generally they feel good, if they are physically fit, mentally alert why stop? I think we are getting more respect because people see how capable, and I am not talking me personally, but generally in the bigger world there are so many at that age group still doing a fantastic job and a lot to offer.
>
> (Chloe)

Similarly, Angela suggests, 'so if you can keep the right weight, eat right and whatever then you can participate in a lot more things and stay active. Not die in a heap when you get to 70. I am trying to do that'.

Despite the association between active lifestyles and health, good health was not a precondition for Sophie's experience engaging in cosmetic surgery and constitution of an 'active' and 'young old' subjectivity. In our interview, Sophie talked about having a near death experience, a chronic condition, cancer and other health problems. At the time I spoke with her Sophie had decided not to undergo any further cosmetic procedures because her post-surgical recovery was becoming too difficult. However, prior to that, her health difficulties had not prevented her from having cosmetic procedures to enhance her appearance and 'feel better'. From these excerpts it is possible to say that rather than good health per se, it is engaging in practices to take care of oneself that is the condition of possibility that enables the constitution of an active lifestyle and the 'young old' subject.

As cultural theorists in ageing studies have observed, the social and cultural constitution of the 'third ager' or 'young old' has occurred through neoliberal and consumer discourses of active, successful, productive and healthy ageing (Featherstone, 1995; Gilleard & Higgs, 2000; Katz & Laliberte-Rudman, 2005; Katz & Marshall, 2003; Powell, 2006; also refer to the Introduction). As Katz (2005: 121) in his article 'Busy Bodies' observes, 'the notion of activity, a recurring motif in popular treatises on longevity since the Enlightenment, today serves as an antidote to pessimistic stereotypes of decline and dependency'. He goes on to argue that modern gerontology and associated healthcare professions have seized on 'activity' as an ethical keyword to generate 'critical intersections between activity and regimens of care and lifestyle with a focus on the management of everyday life in old age'. 'Activity' thus 'marks an alliance between political and personal aspirations' (Cardona, 2008: 481) for 'positive, healthy, independent lives' (Katz, 2005: 126). 'Older' subjectivities styled in relation to principles of being 'active' thus form at the intersection of relations of power (governmentality) and practices of self-care (ethics).

The problem, Katz (2005: 122) argues, is that social welfare policies are eroded in favour of 'neoliberal policies and market-driven programs to "empower" older individuals to be active in order to avoid the stigma and risks of dependency'. However, these policies fail to address the ways in which socio-economic position, gender and race affect the capacity of individuals to engage in practices of self-care and exclude possibilities of 'successful ageing' that are not premised on an individual's ability to be physically and financially independent. 'Ageing well' thus becomes an individual responsibility within a context of structural constraint (Katz and Laliberte-Rudman, 2005: 140–144).

That said, however, 'Deploying a catch-all cry against neoliberalism and governmentality' to show how the 'older' body is 'rendered fodder for the machine that produces "better citizens"' would be, to borrow from Probyn (2008: 402–403), 'the spectacular analysis of the obvious'. In terms of fat and feminism, she argues that whilst this critique proves an obvious point, such scholarship does little to intervene. Like Probyn's critique of feminism, the ageing studies scholarship described, is informed by a narrow reading of Foucault. This means that the insights derived from this work are methodologically and politically limited because they fail to acknowledge agency in terms of the ways 'older' subjectivities are navigated, adapted, adopted and constituted by the subject. The new 'young old' subject, to parallel Gill's (2008: 438–439) argument in relation to postfeminist femininity, 'highlights the way in which power and ideology operate through the construction of subjects, not through top-down imposition but through negotiation, mediation, resistance and articulation'. Rather than simply a governmental practice conditioned by discourses of 'active ageing', I argue that cosmetic surgery can be interpreted as an ethical practice of critique.

Exceeding the boundaries of 'older': cosmetic surgery as an ethical practice of critique

Through critical examination of 'anti-ageing' discourse and the ethics and politics of 'ageing gracefully' the chapters of this book have problematized the conflation of 'ageing' with 'older'. The discussion has demonstrated, as Tulle (2008: 7) suggests, that the problem lies with age acting as a limiting 'structure guiding our social location and our dispositions'. As Dr Wilson observes:

> age is a number and it's a number that society has created to control, you know, maybe for ranking, whatever it is but I think, you know, in the twenty-first century people are living longer and longer…I don't know, age is a number. Age is truly a number, you know.

Dr Wilson might have said that 'age is only a number' but his statement still suggests that chronological age does not confer an essentialist nature to 'older'. Interestingly, Dr Wilson states 'but I honestly, I don't judge people by their age. I don't look at the numeric numbers. I look at their phenotype age.' What Dr Wilson is suggesting by 'phenotype' age implies a judgement based on physical appearance and self-expression and thus the possibility of exceeding limitations imposed by chronological age through self-stylization.

Many of the texts generated for this book suggested that 'age is just a number' and 'old' is a state of mind. Heather for instance proclaims:

> Look I used to nurse with people who were 16 going on 100 who were boring farts and I nursed someone who was 85 going on 16. It's a number. It's all to do with the mind and keeping the body active.

Similarly, Mandy states:

> When you say an age 65 or more people think of you as being a senior citizen, you are old. But really your age is just a number and some people are younger at 65 than others.

Both Dr Smith and James described 'old' as a state of mind unconnected to chronological age:

> I mean I've got patients who are old at forty-five and I've got patients who are young at ninety. Mainly, often it's a mental attitude, I think. You know, if someone's wanting to be interested in life and doing things and out and about and, you know, interacting with whatever club and having some hobbies and sport or whatever, then they're younger than a person who sits at home and does nothing.
>
> (Dr Smith)

> If you are active and healthy then you don't look upon yourself as old, then growing old is a state of mind, because you don't look upon yourself as being old. Whereas you could be 60 and semi invalid and you would consider yourself to be old at 60 and it is a state of mind, because you are not old but you consider yourself to be old.
>
> (James)

Whilst, James' statement reaffirms the importance of health to the subjective experience of 'older', the point is that poor health is not an essential nature of 'older'. A number of texts have problematized the relationship between chronological age and health status, as the following example illustrates through the statement, 'nowadays we often see older people who are fitter and healthier than someone in their 40s, and there is no reason why they should not have surgery' (PanipatOnline.com, 2005).

According to many of the texts, 'older people' are challenging normative expectations in relation to chronological age and transforming what it means to be 'older'. In our interview Chris states:

> Probably these days I would agree 65 is the new 50 if you like. People who are 65 now are probably more able to relate to 50 year olds and their music and what they like to see and what they like to do than maybe

> 65 years olds did 25 years ago. There is better health in older people now than there used to be. The days of you working until you were 60, and dead by the time you were 63, well now you work until you are 70 and you are not dead until you are 83. I don't know how you calculate that, but I don't consider myself an old 70 year old. I consider myself an under 60 year old because of what I like to do which is in part what I have been doing all my life. I don't want to sit around playing cards or snap or bowling and stuff like that. I like jumping out of aeroplanes, once!

Chris' suggestion that '65 is the new 50' reveals a contemporary shift in Western cultures of 'older'. As his statement illustrates, this shift is partly attributable to increasing longevity and accompanying social changes. However, the choice to skydive rather than play cards or bowls speaks to 'older' in terms of new possibilities and practices.

Ms Taylor and Ms Robinson talked about possibilities and practices concerning 'older' in the following statements:

> I think over the last, probably twenty years, there's been more emphasis on keeping yourself looking good and, you know, keeping yourself fit and eating healthy and all those sorts of things, not going grey when you're sixty which is what my grandparents' generation did. Whereas my parents' generation don't seem to do that. They're very active and doing things still. I think that there will be more and more facelifts.
>
> (Ms Taylor)

> I think it's, well they're a lot fitter, I think than my grandparents would have been because they have been taking care of the outside which takes care of the inside, the spirit, which is what nurtures us really and our wellbeing. In essence. If your spirit's good then physically we're good, aren't we? Because you can go out and do that dance, you can go out and you know, do salsa dancing at seventy. You are able to do it. Because you feel good about yourself.
>
> (Ms Robinson)

As these excerpts suggest, these new possibilities and practices are connected to an 'active' lifestyle and regimen of self-care.

Given that 'care of the self' entails critical reflection, Rabinow (2003: 10) observes that it is 'also a form of critique, a critique of the self that entailed perpetual self examination'. Such a critique entails reflection on how we are disciplined with respect to our identities and courses of action in order to test the limits of these forms of subjectivity and relations of power (Gabardi, 2001). Moreover, as Lloyd (1996: 250) argues, 'self-fashioning, *when allied to critique*, can produce sites of contestation over the meanings and contours of identity, and over the ways in which certain practices are mobilized'.

Using Foucault's work on ethics, this chapter has focused on how the practice of cosmetic surgery is reflexively mobilized as a critique of the limits of 'older' subjectivities. Through ethical practices of self-care and self-stylization of active selves and lifestyles, 'older' people are 'challenging dominant discursive representations of old age as burden and decline and reasserting old age as opportunity and choice' (Cardona, 2008: 480). Through ethical self-stylization, spaces of freedom are opened up allowing a creative fashioning of the aesthetic sensibilities that constitute 'older' in ways that exceed the boundaries of ageist discourses.

Rather than a universalist ethics, these practices speak to a relation between the subject and truth that belongs to an aesthetic ethics – an art of 'older' rather than an essential nature. In terms of his own politics and practices, Foucault suggests 'We don't have to discover that we are homosexuals… Rather, we have to create a gay life. To *become*' (Foucault, 1994: 163). Certainly, as we grow older we don't have to discover that we are 'old' or 'elderly' but rather have to create an 'older' life. This brings us back to Foucault's (2005: 109) suggestion quoted in the introduction.

> Old age should not be seen merely as a limit on life, any more than it is to be seen as a phrase of diminished life. Old age should be considered, rather, as a goal, and as a positive goal of existence. We should strive towards old age and not resign ourselves to having it come upon us one day. Old age, with its own forms and values should orient the whole course of life.

With its own 'forms and values' 'older' might be reconceptualized as a telos, a way of being, characteristic of a life well lived. *Becoming* 'older' would thus become a positive goal of existence to be strived towards and reflexively stylized. As Bauman (2008: 125) suggests, 'we are all artists of our lives' and:

> To practice the art of life, to make one's life a 'work of art', amounts in our liquid modern world to being in a state of permanent transformation, to perpetually self-redefine through becoming (or at least trying to become) someone other than one has been thus far.
>
> (Bauman, 2008: 73)

Cosmetic surgery engaged by 'older people' can therefore be reimagined as a practice engaged in the pursuit of *becoming* 'older' rather than denying ageing.

Summary

This chapter explored the ways in which the subjective experience of 'older' is reflexively fashioned amid a cultural politics of 'older' and how cosmetic surgery practice is engaged in pursuit of certain aesthetic values and stylistic criteria. In particular, the ethical and aesthetic principles of 'ageing gracefully' and 'mutton dressed as lamb' were identified and problematized in terms of ageing norms, essentialist discourses of 'natural' ageing and aesthetic practices of self-care. A cultural politics premised on 'ageing gracefully' is therefore limited by the essentialism of the natural body and will fail to transform the discursive framework that renders 'older' bodies undesirable. To overcome this problem, the chapter suggested problematizing 'youth' in aesthetics and developing a (re)inscription of 'older' bodies through desire and desirability. Drawing on participants' discourse to pose a counter politics of 'ageing *dis*-gracefully' drew attention to the ways in which discourses can be seized in acts of voluntary insubordination to modes of subjection that constitute 'older'. The central contention that 'older' people want to look *better* not younger was further developed by exploring the ethical self-stylization of 'older' selves and lifestyles. This is more than an aesthetic preference and is embedded in interpersonal relations between self and other and struggles around subjectivity to challenge, resist and subvert forms of subjectivity connected to being 'aged'. This chapter demonstrates that through creative self- fashioning of aesthetic sensibilities 'older' is being opened up to new possibilities and practices in the context of contemporary ethopolitics that exceed the boundaries of ageist discourses.

Notes

1 Parts of this chapter were published as an article: Garnham, B. (2013). A Cutting Critique: Transforming 'Older' through Cosmetic Surgery. *Ageing & Society*, 34(8), pp.1356–1379. Reprinted with permission from Cambridge University Press.
2 Whether or not beautiful celebrities considered to be 'ageing gracefully' have undergone cosmetic surgery has become a source of fascination and endless speculation in popular media (for one example see Cosmetic Surgery Australia: http://www.cosmeticsurgeryaustralia.com.au/cosmeticcelebrity.htm). Determining whether they are worthy of the admiration associated with the ethical virtues of 'ageing naturally' is therefore a continual ethical dilemma.
3 The photos were taken by Donigan Cumming with consent and active participation.
4 Despite technological development cosmetic surgery is still associated with creating undesirable corporeal forms considered 'plastic' and 'unnatural'.
5 Julia Twigg's work provides further insight into age, ageing and clothing. See Twigg, 2007; Twigg, 2010; Twigg, 2012; Twigg, 2015.

References

Ahmed, S. 2004. *The Cultural Politics of Emotion.* Edinburgh: Edinburgh University Press.

Alphamaleblog. 2006. *Cosmetic Surgery for the Elderly* [Online]. Available: www.alphamaleblog.com/cosmetic-surgery-for-the-elderly.html [Accessed 13 March 2008].

Bauman, Z. 2008. *The Art of Life.* Cambridge: Polity Press.

Besley, T. A. C. & Peters, M. A. 2007. *Subjectivity and Truth: Foucault, Education and the Culture of the Self.* New York: Peter Lang Publishing.

Bildtgård, T. 2000. The Sexuality of Elderly People on Film – Visual Limitations. *Journal of Aging and Identity*, 5, 169–183.

Brown, J. 2006. 'I'm 85 and Still Love Plastic Surgery'. *Women's Day*. Australian Consolidated Press.

Cardona, B. 2008. 'Healthy Ageing' Policies and Anti-ageing Ideologies and Practices: On the Exercise of Responsibility. *Medicine, Health Care and Philosophy*, 11, 475–483.

Daniels, N. 2002. So What's Wrong With Wrinkles? *The Times*.

Elliot, C. 2003. *Better than Well: American Medicine Meets the American Dream*. New York: W.W. Norton & Company.

Featherstone, M. 1995. Post-Bodies, Aging and Virtual Reality. In: Featherstone, M. & Wernick, A. (eds) *Images of Aging: Cultural Representations of Later Life*. London: Routledge.

Foucault, M. 1990. *The Use of Pleasure: The History of Sexuality Volume 2*. USA: Vintage Books.

Foucault, M. 1994. Sex, Power and the Politics of Identity. In: Rabinow, P. (ed.) *Michel Foucault: Ethics, Subjectivity and Truth*. New York: The New Press.

Foucault, M. 1997. What is Critique? In: Lotringer, S. & Hochroth, L. (eds) *The Politics of Truth*. USA: The MIT Press.

Foucault, M. 2005. *The Hermeneutics of the Subject: Lectures at the College De France 1981–1982*. New York: Picador.

Gabardi, W. 2001. *Negotiating Postmodernism*. Minneapolis: University of Minnesota Press.

Gill, R. 2008. Culture and Subjectivity in Neoliberal and Postfeminist Times. *Subjectivity*, 25, 432–445.

Gilleard, C. & Higgs, P. 2000. *Cultures of Ageing: Self, citizen and the body*, Essex, Prentice Hall.

Gilleard, C. & Higgs, P. 2002. The Third Age: Class, Cohort or Generation? *Ageing & Society*, 22, 369–382.

Gilleard, C. & Higgs, P. 2013. *Key Issues in Modern Sociology: Ageing, Corporeality and Embodiment*. London: Anthem Press.

Grove, V. 2000. 'Under The Knife I Find The Real Me'. *The Times*, 26 February.

Hepworth, M. 2003. Ageing Bodies: Aged by Culture. In: Coupland, J. & Gwyn, R. (eds) *Discourse, the Body and Identity*. Hampshire: Palgrave Macmillan.

Hurd Clarke, L. & Griffin, M. 2007. The Body Natural and the Body Unnatural: Beauty Work and Aging. *Journal of Aging Studies*, 21, 187–201.

Katz, S. 2005. Busy Bodies: Activity, Aging, and the Management of Everyday Life. *Cultural Aging: Life Course, Lifestyle, and Senior Worlds*. Toronto: Broadview Press.

Katz, S. & Laliberte-Rudman, D. 2005. Exemplars of Retirement: Identity and Agency Between Lifestyle and Social Movement. *Cultural Aging: Life Course, Lifestyle, and Senior Worlds*. Toronto: Broadview Press.

Katz, S. & Marshall, B. 2003. New Sex for Old: Lifestyle, Consumerism, and the Ethics of Aging Well. *Journal of Aging Studies*, 17, 3–16.

Kornblum, J. 2004. 'I Wanted To Look Like I Feel'. *USA Today*.

Lloyd, M. 1996. A Feminist Mapping of Foucauldian Politics. In: Hekman, S. J. (ed.) *Feminist Interpretations of Michel Foucault*. Pennsylvania: The Pennsylvania State University Press.

Makemeheal.com. 2007. *Under The Plastic Surgery Microscope: Mirren, Streep & Dench* [Online]. Available: http://news.makemeheal.com/helen-mirren-judi-dench-plastic-surgery/79 [Accessed 9 November 2009].

Murray, S. 2005. (Un/Be)Coming Out? Rethinking Fat Politics. *Social Semiotics*, 15, 153–163.

Norris, M. 2003. 60 Years of Plastic Surgery – But Her Love Is Blind. *Women's Day*.

Panipatonline.com. 2005. *New Bodies for Old Souls* [Online]. Available: www.panipatonline.com/article_read.asp?id=1896 [Accessed 13 March 2008].

Potera, C. 2000. *Turning Back Time: New Face, New Outlook* [Online]. Available: www.medicinenet.com/script/main/art.asp?articlekey=51503 [Accessed 13 March 2008].

Powell, J. L. 2006. *Social Theory and Aging*. USA: Rowman & Littlefield Publishers.

Powell, J. L. & Longino, C. F. 2001. Towards the Postmodernization of Aging: The Body and Social Theory. *Journal of Aging and Identity*, 6, 199–207.

Probyn, E. 2008. Silences behind the Mantra: Critiquing Feminist Fat. *Feminism & Psychology*, 18, 401–404.

Rabinow, P. 2003. *Anthropos Today: Reflections on Modern Equipment*. New Jersey: Princeton University Press.

Robotham, J. 2004. Boomers Keep Raising Eyebrows. *Sydney Morning Herald*.

Ryan, D. 2001. Adding Years Gracefully. *The Age*.

Shilling, C. 2003. *The Body and Social Theory*. London: Sage Publications.

Stock, R. W. 1996. Senior Class: Face-Lift Surgery Gains Adherents. *The New York Times*, 25 July.

The CanadianPress. 2002. More People 65 and Older Getting Cosmetic Surgery. 24 July.

Tulle-Winton, E. 2000. Old Bodies. In: Hancock, P., Hughes, B., Jagger, E., Paterson, K., Russell, R., Tulle-Winton, E. & Tyler, M. (eds) *The Body, Culture and Society: An Introduction*. Buckingham: Open University Press.

Tulle, E. 2008. The Ageing Body and the Ontology of Ageing: Athletic Competence in Later Life. *Body & Society*, 14, 1–19.

Tulloch, L. 2004. Facing the Future. *Australian Women's Weekly*, November.

Turner, B. S. 1995. Aging and Identity: Some Reflections on the Somatization of the Self. In: Featherstone, M. & Wernick, A. (eds) *Images of Aging: Cultural Representations of Later Life*. London: Routledge.

Twigg, J. 2004. The body, Gender, and Age: Feminist Insights in Social Gerontology. *Journal of Aging Studies*, 18, 59–73.

Twigg, J. 2007. Clothing, Age and the Body: A Critical Review. *Ageing & Society*, 27, 285–305.

Twigg, J. 2010. Clothing and Dementia: A Neglected Dimension? *Journal of Aging Studies*, 24, 223–230.

Twigg, J. 2012. Adjusting the Cut: Fashion, the Body and Age on the UK High Street. *Ageing and Society*, 32, 1030–1054.

Twigg, J. 2015. Dress and Age: The Intersection of Life and Work. *International Journal of Ageing and Later Life*, 10, 55–67.

Vares, T. 2009. Reading the 'Sexy Oldie': Gender, Age(ing) and Embodiment. *Sexualities*, 12, 503–524.

Weiss, D. & Kukla, R. 2009. The 'Natural Look': Extreme Makeovers and the Limits of Self-Fashioning. In: Heyes, C. & Jones, M. (eds) *Cosmetic Surgery: A Feminist Primer*. Surrey: Ashgate Publishing.

6 Concluding cuts

This book aims to 'de-territorialize' (Braidotti, 2002) 'older' from normative discourses of ageing. Beginning with the embodied 'older' self engaged in a practice of body modification, this ambition is pursued through a nuanced descriptive, ethical and political reading of 'older' identity politics nested within the contemporary ethico-political terrain of self-care. Ethically sensitive and theoretically attuned to statements with political momentum, this approach provides insight into the wilful reformation of discourses at an early stage of their transformation emerging from a 'virtual fracture' (Foucault, 1988a: 36) in the politics of truth. Statements such as '*designing* older rather than denying ageing', 'to look *better* not younger' and 'ageing *dis*gracefully' exceed semantic differentiation. Indeed, they direct us toward transgressive possibilities that rupture the system of thought that has hitherto oppressed the constitution of the 'older' subject. This wilful reformation of discourse provides evidence of an active cultural politics of 'older' emerging from the critically reflexive engagement of older people with cosmetic surgery. The argument of this book is that this engagement constitutes a 'cutting critique' of 'ageing' discourses enmeshed in an aesthetic mode of subjectivation that underpins a 'new ethics of old age' (Foucault, 1994a: 110).

Troubling ageing

Discourses of ageing have been relentlessly pursued, hailed and critically questioned throughout the chapters of this book, as the trouble with 'older' and the object to be troubled. It's not that I would contend that we must rid ourselves of ageing or that ageing has nothing to contribute to understanding the ontology of the subject. My concerns are historicized and situated in terms of the cultural geographies of ageing that have colonized 'older' and enacted an oppressive, stigmatizing and constrictive regimen of 'truth' that provides the foundation for ageism. The chapters of this book provide textual evidence that normative discourses of ageing inscribe pathological decline, decrepitude and risk in the corporeality of 'older', fracture 'older' subjectivity, sustain 'youthful' ideals of appearance, identity and lifestyle, and render cosmetic surgery an 'anti-ageing' practice connected to an ageist culture. In this discursive framework, cosmetic surgery becomes anathema to the cultural politics of 'ageing naturally' which entails acceptance and display of the 'naturally' ageing body. As the texts analysed in Chapter 5 suggest however, 'ageing gracefully' is deemed to necessitate the stylization of 'older' in ways deemed 'age appropriate'. This colonization of 'older' by the 'true' discourses of 'natural ageing' therefore delimits the stylization of 'older' selves and lifestyles in ways that are aesthetically, ethically, socially, culturally and politically restrictive and potentially oppressive for *becoming* 'older'.

Whilst ageing norms exert power to shape the ethical stylization of 'older', they are also problematized and unsettled by older people who undergo cosmetic surgery. This is because, as a practice of body modification, cosmetic surgery has the potential to reshape 'ageing' norms, but more importantly, transform the discursive system that maintains their boundaries (also see Gilleard and Higgs, 2013). For instance, the increased visibility and stylization of the 'older' body may begin to rupture the normative binary structured discourses of 'youthfulness' and 'agedness'. Through the problematization and transformation of the discursive framework that normalizes 'youthful' aesthetic ideals, a greater freedom and acceptance of the 'older' body might be attained with its attendant de-stigmatization and selective valorization. Indeed, an aesthetic connected to desirable 'older' bodies may emerge that problematizes beauty and ageing. I believe such an aesthetic already occupies contemporary cultural spaces and whilst being easily recognizable upon presentation, is largely ignored by academic critics. That beauty and aesthetics offer transgressive appeal emerges because 'beauty always exceeds the rule that defines it' (Holliday and Taylor, 2006: 180).

Of course, this is a controversial position to assume and will be critically problematized in terms of its foundations in 'beauty', 'freedom' and 'agency'. I would like therefore, to emphasize that in taking up this position I am not uncritically asserting a new arrangement of norms to prefigure ethical and aesthetic sensibilities. As Foucault (1991: 84) argued, the practice of critique 'should be an instrument for those who fight, those who resist and refuse what is…It doesn't have to lay down the law for the law. It isn't a stage in a programming. It's a challenge directed to what is.' Foucault and those that follow his methodology have been critiqued for 'failing' to provide normative grounds for their critical analyses. Given this critique has been levelled at her own work, Butler provides a response by first asking 'under what political conditions does possibility itself emerge as a political good?' She answers, 'under conditions in which gender has been constrained, in which certain sexual and gender minorities have felt their lives to be "impossible", unviable, unlivable, then "becoming possible" is a most certain political achievement' (Butler and Connolly, 2000: 7–8). Whilst I do not intend for the comparison to be overworked, certain parallels can be drawn here. The position advanced by this book is strategic given the merit of deconstructing the system of 'truth' connected to 'ageing' for a cultural politics that provides creative possibilities for 'older' identities, bodies, values and lifestyles that give form to a desirable old age. Given the modern history in which 'older' people have been subject to cultural invisibility, marginalization and stigmatization, this is a worthy endeavour and 'becoming possible' within mainstream consumer society and culture is a desirable political achievement.

The political reading presented here is also sympathetic to Foucault's (1994b: 231–232) assertion:

> My point is not that everything is bad, but that everything is dangerous, which is not exactly the same as bad. If everything is dangerous, then we always have something to do. So my position leads not to apathy but to a hyper- and pessimistic activism.

As cultural gerontologists have argued, the neoliberal political rationalities and practices of consumption that support the contemporary ethics of self-care pose dangers for *becoming* 'older'. This is because whilst neoliberalism places ethical demands on the subject for self-care, its structures do not necessarily provision individuals with the economic, cultural and social resources needed to ensure care, and disciplinary practices of normalizing power may render outside positions for those whose ageing is not 'positive', 'successful' or 'active' difficult, distressing or even unliveable. However, as the analyses presented in this book have demonstrated, these arguments would benefit from further examination based on more nuanced analyses of older people's experiences navigating the discursive terrain of self-care and the cultural politics of 'older'. For instance, Chapter 5 illustrates that health and wealth, often cited as preconditions for 'successful ageing', did not exclude older participants with illness and limited income who desired engagement with care of the self and stylization of a desirable appearance and social identity. Moreover, as Gilleard and Higgs (2013: 166) suggest:

> The desire to look good, to feel good and to be good need not be devalued because these goals can never be fully individually realized. Taking care of oneself by taking care of one's body is not obviously motivated by a wish to deprive others of such opportunities, nor is it motivated by a desire to render others weaker, sicker or uglier. The desire to live better longer cannot be opposed on the grounds that not all will succeed or because such goals can never be permanently realized.

Within the current conditions of possibility that constitute the ethico-political domain, taking care of the self to look and feel good is a reasonable life strategy for whom its practitioners should not be met with derision and derogation for 'denying ageing'. Indeed, I believe that the participants interviewed for this book have provided a valuable insight into a far deeper critique of 'ageing' than has hitherto been recognized by scholarship in this field.

It is a central contention of this book that critical ageing studies and cultural gerontology would benefit from engagement with Foucault's work on ethics to understand 'older' people's experiences and engagement with practices of self-care. For too long it has been the habit of the critical ageing studies literature to be restricted by a dominance of perspectives in which the operation of disciplinary power on bodies constitutes a privileged focus for critical inquiry. Whilst this scholarship has provided ethically and politically important critiques by rendering visible the operation of bio-power, it has been insensible to the generative capacity of bodies and agency of thinking subjects operating in a micro-politics from which a wellspring of discursive resistance, transgression and transformation might emerge. Foucault's work has provided a lens for a nuanced account of the operation of power, a framework for analysing the contemporary ethico-political domain and the production of 'older' subjectivities, and an ethical and political impetus through critique. However, it has been the textual data that has provided the discursive resources and strategies of resistance that have shaped the arguments proposed in each of the chapters. Drawing on a 'reasoned cartography' as 'the starting point for the production of adequate accounts of the realities involved', this book has therefore pursued 'the quest for resistance' as its 'ultimate aim' (Braidotti, 2002: 265).

Becoming 'older'

In addition to its problematization of normative discourses of ageing, this book has offered an approach to theorizing *becoming* 'older'. It is a strategic approach that provides possibilities for understanding that 'older' subjectivities are 'about affinities and the capacity both to sustain and generate inter-connectedness' (Braidotti, 2002: 8). Rather than 'pinned down by the category "old"' (Cruikshank, 2013: 6), the participants interviewed for this book demonstrate agentic capacity to navigate, resist, take up and transform reasoned discourses to stylize self-identity within the conditions of possibility and cultural practices available to them. This agentic capacity flows from desire as the guiding and productive force to *becoming* that establishes affinities and the inter-connectedness of the subject with the 'assemblages' of 'older'. As Braidotti (2002: 71) elaborates, 'the construction of a thinking subject cannot be separated from that of a desiring subject…the key idea here is that desire is the first and foremost step in the process of constitution of a self'.

As a theoretical approach with a political sensibility, becoming 'older' operates strategically to transgress the boundaries of the normative discursive framework of 'ageing'. However, this system also requires critical intervention and problematization in terms of creative possibilities for inscribing 'ageing' back into the ontology of 'older'. This is theoretically important since 'ageing' provides the temporal pathway to *becoming* 'older'. It is intriguing to consider the possibilities afforded by thinking through 'becoming' to consider the ontology of ageing. If 'becoming' evokes a continuous flow then perhaps ageing can be considered a temporal dimension to embodied subjectivity, one that encapsulates a personal history, corporeal changes, memories of lived experience and a simultaneously continued and transformative sense of selfhood. Baars work in cultural gerontology is leading advances in this thinking through her problematization of 'chronometric age', or calendar age, as a restrictive discourse that limits our understanding of 'what it means to *live in time*' (Baars, 2012: 5, emphasis in original). She argues for the need to develop an existential dimension to ageing; one that engages with an art of ageing and narrative identity that provide a site for the enmeshment of 'socio-cultural macro-narratives and personal experiences' (Baars, 2012: 8). The discourses that emerge from this form of problematization will provide the resources needed to inscribe the lacuna of meaning offered by the 'simulacrum of agelessness' (Gilleard and Higgs, 2013: 166). However, it remains theoretically, politically and ethically important to ensure that ageing does not re-colonize 'older' through an assault on this front, because the ontological possibilities presented by 'older' exceed those of ageing.

A new ethic of 'older': politics of performativity

This book poses and provides textual evidence of a 'new ethics of old age' (Foucault, 1994a: 110). It presents the contemporary 'aestheticization of everyday life' as a stylistics of existence in which aesthetic and ethical principles operate to constitute 'desirable'[1] forms and values for being 'older'. In this context 'older' is produced through practices of *becoming* as expressions of agency and self-stylization. Through this rendition, 'older' bodies are desiring bodies and the freedom to engage in diverse practices generates possibilities for a multiplicity of 'older' subjectivities. As Gilleard and Higgs (2013: 164) suggest

> rather than being enslaved by youth or made subject to the tyranny of old age, the body can be approached as always more open than this, an inexorably polysemous vehicle that allows for the expression of multiple lifestyles that can be realized and modified at different times and in points in the lifecycle.

Beginning to think about the creative possibilities proffered by becoming 'older' will enable new insights that further problematize taken for granted assumptions. Sandberg's (2013) work on affirmative old age in the context of sexuality and ageing masculinity for instance, is instructive in this regard. Through participant narratives and feminist theories of embodied difference, Sandberg's analysis illuminates new and unforeseen possibilities for desire and sexual experience that problematize discourses of functional loss or threat to masculine identity.

Gilleard and Higgs (2013: 161) rightly assert that the contemporary phenomena, that they term, 'new ageing', has emerged in resistance to 'not becoming old' – when old is stripped of agency, choice and cultural desirability. However, it is less about 'not becoming old' but rather, 'how not to be governed like that, by that, in the name of those principles, with such and such an objective in mind and by means of such procedures, not like that, not for that, not by them' (Foucault, 1984a: 28). This is why *becoming* older offers a strategic critical imperative to recognize the stylization of desirable 'older' subjectivities. This approach need not assert new normative binaries between 'successfully and unsuccessfully ageing bodies' (Gilleard and Higgs, 2013: 165). Systems of thought that constitute old age as a lifestage burdened by vulnerability and dependency and 'successful' ageing as a strategy for staving off inevitable decline for as long as possible require problematization to illuminate the ways in which human vulnerabilities, dependencies and needs are dynamic and wax and wane across the lifecourse. Rather, the political intent of *becoming* 'older' is aligned to 'queering', such that difference and its proliferation are freed from normative and disciplinary systems.

The analysis presented in this book suggests that 'older' people who engage in cosmetic surgery practise ethical critique. A critique that entails 'a moment of ethical questioning' that 'poses the question anew: who will be a subject here, and what will count as a life' (Butler, 2001: 20). As Chapter 5 demonstrates, the 'rejection of an imposed identity and a set of norms becomes the impetus for fashioning one's own ethical code and conduct' (Gabardi, 2001: 78–79). This means that the 'taken-for-granted can change', as Rabinow (2003: 67 citing Racjman, 1996) observes, because:

> When this mode becomes reflexive, it becomes an aesthetic "not of taste nor of beautiful appearance but of the invention of new sensibilities, new concepts, new techniques and ideas of technique in response to those incommensurabilities that question our practices and that eventualize our relation to them".

An aesthetic mode of subjectivation thus enables the modification and transformation of 'older' sensibilities. The political implications of the practice of ethical critique is elaborated by Gabardi (2001: 78–79) who writes:

> freedom entails a movement from resistance to ethics to political action. Resistance, the most primal expression of freedom, involves the revolt of the body against the normalizing effects of disciplinary power. This critical resistance, largely reactive and defensive is channeled into an affirmative ethical project concerned with self-care…The ethical agent becomes a political actor in joining struggles that seek to alter power relations so that one can more freely live one's life. The battle is joined at the local and microlevels by countering norms with norms and techniques with techniques.

The transformation of 'older' through ethical practices of self-care is therefore a struggle to alter relations of power and exceed the boundaries of 'ageing' so that 'one can more freely live one's life'. Acts of 'voluntary insubordination', captured by the cultural politics of 'ageing *dis*gracefully', operate to detach 'the power of truth from the forms of hegemony, social, economic, and cultural, within which it operates at the present time' (Foucault, 1984b: 74–75). As Foucault (1988b: 155) observes, 'as soon as one can no longer think things as one formerly thought them, transformation becomes both very urgent, very difficult, and quite possible'.

The theoretical, analytic and political discourses that constitute this book inaugurate its own limitations and constraints. To problematize ageing and the ontology of 'older' as its central focus and concern, this book brackets out questions of how place, race, class, gender and sexuality intersect and complicate the formation of 'older' subjectivities. Given the traditional neglect of ageing by feminist theorists of intersectionality and the parallel neglect of intersectional subjectivities within gerontology and ageing studies, much work is needed to elaborate these lines of inquiry (see Calasanti and King, 2015). In addition, by focusing on 'older' people who have undergone cosmetic surgery, this book also privileges aesthetic concerns regarding the stylization of the 'older' body. These concerns were of direct theoretical and analytic relevance to this book. However, this does not suggest that these are immediate concerns held by all 'older' people or that these concerns are foundational to the cultural politics of 'older'. Whilst the practice of cosmetic surgery enables 'older' people to re-claim, re-design and re-inscribe their bodies in ways that transfigure the limitations of ageing and ageist discourses, transformation is not restricted to cosmetic surgery or even aesthetic body modification practices. For instance, Marshall and Rahman's (2015: 580) work suggests that 'A key aspect of ageing fandom is the legitimization of transformations in age norms that ageing celebrity can provide.' This work seeks to explore:

> the contributions of celebrity culture to the construction of new forms of ageing identity, challenging and transforming traditional assumptions about the infirmities of body and mind, the lack of cultural engagement and the lack of technological *savoir faire* in the older generation.
>
> (Marshall and Rahman, 2015: 580)

What this suggests is that celebrity culture is providing a 'surface of emergence' (Foucault, 1972) for the problematization of 'older' and transformation of norms. Given their heightened visibility, media driven cultures are a privileged site for the cultural politics of 'older'. However, scholarship that explores and illuminates these transformations also constitutes a surface of emergence for discourses of 'older' and 'ageing' and thus is central to this political project. This is why research practices that ethically engage the cultural politics of 'older' are needed to generate new and modified knowledges that render 'older' intelligible in ways that allow for complexity, contradictions and creative possibilities. This book accomplishes elements of such a transformative enterprise through a case study that reinscribes 'older' and the practice of cosmetic surgery. It is a 'performative' text that produces a cultural politics of 'older' as the object of its discourse, the very thing of which it speaks. In doing so, it provides a surface of emergence for new and modified discourses that can be seized and deployed in strategies to drive social and cultural change.

The transformative possibilities developed in this book suggest that things can always be 'otherwise'. However, the cartographic practices used to map conditions of possibility do not aim

> to destabilize the present by pointing to its contingency, but to destabilize the future by recognizing its openness. That is to say, in demonstrating that no single future is written in our present, it might fortify our abilities, in part through thought itself, to intervene in that present, and so to shape something of the future that we might inhabit.
>
> (Rose, 2001: 5)

As an intervention in the present, this book demands change to practice if we are to 'shape something of the future' that we wish to inhabit. One thing is for certain, and that is we are all becoming 'older'. By attending to cultural texts and practices in the present we can shape something of the opportunities and possibilities that 'older' has to offer in the future. Through its themes of *subjectivity, surgery and self-stylization*, this book speaks to the cultural politics of 'older'. It is a book about truth, beauty and freedom.

Note

1 'Desirable' is evoked here not merely to refer to normative appearance/identities but *telos*, the forms and values that are pursued through ethical self-stylization.

References

Baars, J. 2012. *Aging and the Art of Living*. Baltimore, MD: Johns Hopkins University Press.

Braidotti, R. 2002. *Metamorphoses: Towards a Materialist Theory of Becoming*. UK & USA: Polity Press.

Butler, J. 2001. *What is Critique? An Essay on Foucault's Virtue* [Online]. Available: http://www.law.berkeley.edu/centers/kadish/what%20is%20critique%20J%20Butler.pdf [Accessed 30 August 2006].

Butler, J. & Connolly, W. 2000. Politics, Power and Ethics: A Discussion between Judith Butler and William Connolly. *Theory & Event*, 4, 28.

Calasanti, T. & King, N. 2015. Intersectionality and Age. In: Twigg, J. & Martin, W. (eds) *Routledge Handbook of Cultural Gerontology*. Oxon: Routledge.

Cruikshank, M. 2013. *Learning to Be Old: Gender, Culture and Aging*. Plymouth: Rowman & Littlefield.

Foucault, M. 1972. *The Archaeology of Knowledge and the Discourse on Language*. New York: Pantheon Books.

Foucault, M. 1984a. Polemics, Politics, and Problemizations. In: Rabinow, P. (ed.) *The Foucault Reader*. Hamondsworth: Penguin.

Foucault, M. 1984b. Truth and Power. In: Rabinow, P. (ed.) *The Foucault Reader: An Introduction to Foucault's Thought*. New York: Random House.

Foucault, M. 1988a. Critical Theory/Intellectual History. In: Kritzman, L. D. (ed.) *Michel Foucault: Politics, Philosophy, Culture: Interviews and other Writings 1977–1984*. New York: Routledge.

Foucault, M. 1988b. Practicing Criticism. In: Kritzman, L. D. (ed.) *Michel Foucault. Politics, Philosophy, Culture: Interviews and other Writings 1977–1984*. New York: Routledge.

Foucault, M. 1991. Questions of Method. In: Burchell, G., Gordon, C. & Miller, P. (eds) *The Foucault Effect: Studies in Governmentality*. Hertfordshire: Harvester Wheatsheaf.

Foucault, M. 1994a. Nietzsche, Freud, Marx. In: Faubion, J. D. (ed.) *Michel Foucault: Ethics, Subjectivity and Truth*. New York: New York Press.

Foucault, M. 1994b. On the Genealogy of Ethics: An Overview of a Work in Progress. In: Rabinow, P. (ed.) *Michel Foucault: Ethics, Subjectivity and Truth*. New York: The New York Press.

Gabardi, W. 2001. *Negotiating Postmodernism*. Minneapolis: University of Minnesota Press.

Gilleard, C. & Higgs, P. 2013. *Key Issues in Modern Sociology: Ageing, Corporeality and Embodiment*. London: Anthem Press.

Holliday, R. & Taylor, J. 2006. Aesthetic Surgery as False Beauty. *Feminist Theory*, 7, 179–195.

Marshall, B. L. & Rahman, M. 2015. Celebrity, Ageing and the Construction of 'Third Age' Identities. *International Journal of Cultural Studies*, 18, 577–593.

Rabinow, P. 2003. *Anthropos Today: Reflections on Modern Equipment*. New Jersey: Princeton University Press.

Rose, N. 2001. The Politics of Life Itself. *Theory, Culture & Society*, 18(6), 1–30.

Sandberg, L. 2013. Affirmative Old Age: The Ageing Body and Feminist Theories on Difference. *International Journal of Ageing and Later Life*, 8, 11–40.

Index

'abject' 68
active ageing 10
active 'older' self and lifestyle 115–19
Adler, Alfred 89
aesthetic enhancement 21, 79–80
aestheticization of everyday life 6, 130: aged body and 107; creating a lifestyle and 39; self-care and 20, 21, 37, 95; self-knowledge and 37
aesthetics: cosmetic surgery and 93–5; ethics and 34–5; problematizing youth in 106–10
age: chronological 13–14, 58–60, 119–20; as just a number 119–20; social location and 106
age-appropriate appearance 101, 112–13
age-appropriate norms: clothing and 112–13; transgression of 110–11
aged body, social and cultural marginalization of 107–8
age-inappropriateness, cosmetic surgery and 104
ageing: becoming older and 7–8; biomedicalization of 3, 6, 8–9, 11; body and 14–15; Cartesian dualism and essentialist ethic of 61–2; as cultural process 11–12; denying 1–2, 15–16; dissonance in 57–60; mask of 21, 60, 61; natural 79, 99; 'new' 17–18, 130–31; ontology of 12–13; premature 58; preventative intervention for effects of 74–5; reversing effects of 74–5; socio-political regulation of 9–11; successful 11; *see also* 'new' ageing
ageing celebrities 100, 108, 123n2
ageing discourse 2, 30, 126–8
ageing disgracefully 21–2, 99; cultural politics of 110–12
ageing gracefully 22, 99–102, 127; cultural politics of 105–6
ageism: cosmetic surgery and 1–2; feminism and 6
agelessness, simulacrum of 130
agency: *becoming* and 5; body as site for exercising 3–5; cosmetic surgery and 30
age-related norms 13–14, 110–11, 112–13; denying 15–16
Ahmed, S. 101
Angela (study participant): on age-appropriate dressing 112; on being young old 118; on decision to have cosmetic surgery 111; profile of **49**; on risk of cosmetic surgery 67; on self-care 84
anti-ageing discourse 2, 14–15, 21, 30, 73, 75; problematizing 75–9
appearance: age-appropriate 101; aging body's 14–15; dissonance between chronological age and 58–60
authentic self 62–4

Baars, J. 7–8, 129–30
baby boomers, appearance and consumerism and 109–10
Baudrillard, J. 5, 40, 93
Bauman, Z. 5, 39–40, 122
becoming 5, 40–2
becoming 'older' 122, 128, 129–30, 131
Better Than Well (Elliot) 61–2, 86–7
biogerontology 8
biomedicalization of ageing 3, 6, 8–9, 11
blepharoplasty 76
bodily maintenance, self-care and 81–8
body: age, ageing, and appearance of 14–15; as art form 94–5; Cartesian dualism and 61–2; deviant 65–8;

enfolded relation to self 64; in games of truth 57–60; marginalization of aged 107–8; natural 15, 102–5; normative 65–8; power in materiality of 102; as site for exercising agency 3–5; as site for work on self 40; subjectization and 40–2
body modification 4; constitution of self and 64; cosmetic surgery and 31
Bourdieu, P. 13, 106
Braidotti, R. 2, 69, 129
Dr Brown (study participant): on aesthetics and cosmetic surgery 93; on cosmetic surgery and psychological health 88; on cosmetic surgery as consumer practice 90; on looking natural 103–4; on making patients 'more well' 86; on preventing effects of ageing 75; profile of **51**
Butler, Judith: on aesthetic fashioning of the body 95; on folding of force 41; on gender 13; on possibility as political good 127; on power and subjectivation 5; on subject, truth and being 'otherwise' 15–16; on transforming self 45–6

care of the self 35–7; association with narcissism 36–7; critique and 121; lifestyles and 80–92; new ethic of 'older' and 44–6
Cartesian ethics: of ageing 20–1, 61–2; know yourself and 37
celebrities, ageing 100, 108, 123n2
Charlotte (study participant): on active lifestyle and wealth 116; on age and cosmetic surgery 65; on age-appropriate cosmetic surgery 104; on bodily maintenance 82; on cosmetic surgery and psychological health 88; on decision to have cosmetic surgery 111; on dissonance between chronological age and appearance 58; on enhancing appearance through surgery 79; profile of **49**; on reasons older people have cosmetic surgery 68; on transgression of age-appropriate norms 110–11; on treatment of older persons 114
Chloe (study participant): on active lifestyle and wealth 116; on appearance and lifestyles 80–1; on being young old and lifestyle 117–18; on bodily maintenance 82; on cosmetic surgery and psychological health 88; on cosmetic surgery as consumer practice 90; on cosmetic surgery as self-indulgence 91; on dissonance between outer expression and inner feeling 60; profile of **49**; on reasons older people have cosmetic surgery 68; on risks of cosmetic surgery 103; on vanity 81
Chris (study participant): on active lifestyle and wealth, 116; on cosmetic surgery and clothing choices, 113; on cosmetic surgery and psychological health, 88; on cultural shift in 'older,' 120–1; dissonance between inner feelings and appearance to others, 59–60; profile of, **49**
Christian ethics, care of the self and 36
chronological age 13–14, 119–20; dissonance between appearance and 58–60
chrononormativity 14
clothing, age-appropriate norms and 110–11, 112–13
confessional practice, subjectivation and 63
consumer culture: baby boomers and 109–10; cosmetic surgery and 5–6, 21, 87–8; ethopolitics and 37–44; youth and 106
consumer discourses, cosmetic surgery and 89–92
consumer subjectivity 39–40
Dr Cooper (study participant): on age and cosmetic surgery 65–6; on dissonance between chronological age and appearance 58; on looking natural after cosmetic surgery 104; on older patients changing shape 77; on plastic surgery 87; profile of **51**
cosmetic surgeons: challenging authority of 70n1; consultation with patient 63
cosmetic surgery: age-appropriate 104; age categories and use of 76–7; ageism and 1–2; agency and 30; as anti-ageing medicine 15; as autonomous choice 91; becoming a subject and 4–5; blending with leisure 91–2; bodily incongruence and 104; as bodily maintenance 81–8; body modification and 4, 31; Cartesian dualism and 62; changing shape and 77; consumer culture and 5–6, 21; cost of 117; critique of 73; defined 87; dissonance

between chronological age and appearance and 58; as ethical practice of critique 119–22, 131; ethic of creativity and freedom and 93–5; hermeneutics of self and 62–3; to look better, not younger 21, 79–80; normative *vs.* deviant bodies and 65–8; participant profiles **49–50**; passing as natural 102–5; plastic surgery *vs.* 75–6, 87; practices of self and 43, 44–5; practitioner profiles **51–2**; risks of 66–7, 102–5; self-care and 19–20, 21, 73, 81–8; self-fulfillment and 21, 81, 88–9; self-indulgence and 21, 81, 89–92; self-stylization and 2, 19–20, 22
cosmetic surgery clinics, as hybrid spaces 91–2
cosmetic surgery travel industry 92
Crawford, R. 85–6
creativity, cosmetic surgery and 93–5
critical ageing studies 11–13, 128–9
critical ontology of the self 45
critique: cosmetic surgery as ethical practice of 119–22; as ethical practice 112; of 'older' 6–7; practice of 44, 45–6, 127
Cruikshank, M. 6, 7, 13, 17, 67–8
cultural gerontology 12–13
cultural politics: of ageing disgracefully 110–12; of ageing gracefully 105–6
cultural shift in what it means to be 'older' 120–2

dandysm 36, 54n3
Deleuze, G. 41, 42, 43–4
demographic ageing, problem of 1, 10
deviant bodies 65–8
discourse, Foucault on 32, 106; *see also individual discourses*
dissonance: between chronological age and appearance 58–60; between inner feeling and appearance to others 59–60

Elliot, C. 61–2, 89, 103
Emily (study participant): on age-appropriate dressing 112; on dissonance between outer expression and inner feeling 60; profile of **49**
empirical data 46–53; chronology of media texts **47–8**; participant profiles **49–50**; practitioner profiles **51–2**
enhancement technologies, medicine *vs.* 87
ethical critique, cosmetic surgery as 119–22, 131
ethical principles, aesthetic relationship with self and 34–5
ethical problematization of old age 18–19
ethical substance 42
ethic of 'older,' new 18–22, 130–33; care of self and 44–6
ethics: care of the self and 35–7; essentialist ethic of ageing 61–2; Foucault on 31–5; freedom and 46; 'know yourself' and 35–7; politics as 2; *see also* Cartesian ethics
ethopolitics 2, 37–44

fat body 75
fat politics 105–6
Featherstone, M. 5–6, 39, 91
feelings, dissonance between appearance to others and inner 59–60
feminism: ageism and 6; on cosmetic surgery 4
Foucault, Michel 119; on activism 128; body as signification and 15; care of the self and 19–20, 35–7; on critique as ethical practice 112; ethical substance and 42; hermeneutics of the subject and 62, 63–4; on interpretation 53; 'know yourself' and 35–7; mode of subjection and 42; on old age 20, 122; on power 5, 129; power in materiality of the body and 102; on power of truth 132; on practice of critique 127; practices of self and 42–3, 44–6; problematization and 53; on resistance 44; subjectivation and 5, 20, 21, 40–2; *telos* 43–4; on theory 31; writings on ethics 31–5
fracture 62; new ageing as instrument of 69–70
freedom: ethics and 46; self-care and ethic of 93–5

Gabardi, W. 44, 94, 131
games of truth 32, 36; body and subject in 57–60
gerontology, cultural 12–13
Gilleard, C. 18; on ageing as cultural process 12, 17; on anti-ageing medicine 15; on controlling aesthetics of ageing 80; critique of 'older' 6, 7; on focus on poor and disabled elderly 11; on health 86; on lack of problematizing of ageing 69; on living

better longer 128, 130; on resistance to looking aged 113, 114; on signs of ageing and care of self 84–5; on social policies and ageing 9; on staying young culture 107; on third agers 10
Gray Panthers 23n3
Greco-Roman Antiquity: formation of subjectivity and 41–2; practices of the self in 33–4, 35–7; reimagining 'older' and ethics of 20
Grosz, E. 3–4, 64, 65

habitus 106
Ms Harris (study participant): on cosmetic surgery and bodily incongruence 104; on cosmetic surgery as autonomous choice 91; profile of **51**
health: being 'older' and 120–1; being young old and 118; as state of well-being 85–6; will to 86
healthism 85–6
Heather (study participant): on age and cosmetic surgery 65; on age as just a number 120; on bodily maintenance 83; on cosmetic surgery and bodily incongruence 104; on dissonance between outer expression and inner feeling 60; on looking good for one's age 67; profile of **49**; on reasons older people have cosmetic surgery 113; on reversing effects of ageing 74; on vanity 82
The Hermeneutics of the Subject (Foucault) 35, 36, 63
Heyes, C. 4, 70n1, 96n4
Higgs, P. 18; on ageing as cultural process 12, 17; on anti-ageing medicine 15; on controlling aesthetics of ageing 80; critique of 'older' 6, 7; on focus on poor and disabled elderly 11; on lack of problematizing of ageing 69; on living better longer 128, 130; on resistance to looking aged 113, 114; on signs of ageing and care of self 84–5; on social policies and ageing 9; social policy and aging 11; on staying young culture 107; on third agers 10; will to health and 86

identity, true 15–16
identity formation, as project 2–3
identity politics of 'older' 7
individual responsibility, young old concept and 118–19
Isabella (study participant): on being active 115; cost of cosmetic surgery and 117; profile of **50**

James (study participant): on ageing gracefully 99–100, 100–1; on being young old 117; criticism of engaging in anti-ageing practices 78-9; on looking good for one's age 67; on 'old' as state of mind 120; profile of **50**
Jones, M. 4, 5, 70n1, 80, 94

Katz, S. 10, 19, 118–19
know how, responsibility for self and 39
know yourself 35–7

leisure practices, cosmetic surgery and 91–2
lifestyle: ageing and healthy 11; care of self and 80–92; responsibility for social welfare and 39; stylization of active 115–19
liposuction 76
logos 43
looking good for one's age 67–8, 84

makeover culture 5
Mandy (study participant): on age as just a number 120; on cosmetic surgery and clothing choices 113; cost of cosmetic surgery and 117; on decision to have cosmetic surgery 111; notion of 're' and 74; profile of **50**; on risk of cosmetic surgery 66; on vanity 82
marginalization, of aged body 107–8
Ms Martin (study participant) 87; profile of **52**
mask of ageing 21, 60, 61
media, aesthetically ideal images of older body in 108–9
medical tourism 92
medicine, enhancement technologies *vs.* 87
mental health, cosmetic surgery and 88–9
Möbius strip 64
mode of subjection 42
moral action 43
Murray, S. 75, 105, 106
'mutton dressed as lamb' 99–102

natural ageing 79, 99
natural body: ageing and 15; cosmetic surgery and appearance of 102–5
neoliberalism: becoming older and self-care 128; consumerism and 38; ethopolitics and 37–44; social policy and ageing well 18–19; young old and 10–11, 118–19
'new' ageing 17–18, 130–31; fracture and 69–70
normative bodies 65–8

'old,' as state of mind 119–20
'older': becoming 7–8, 16–18, 21–2, 122, 129–30, 131; critique of 6–7; cultural shift in what it means to be 120–2; designing 2
older people: changing shape through cosmetic surgery 77–8; critical truth of 'older' in acts and appearances of 16; increased use of cosmetic surgery 1–2; increased visibility of 1, 109; invisibility of 113–14; powerlessness of 6–7
'older' self: aesthetic stylization of 112–14; Cartesian ethics and 20–1; doing differently 2–6; intersection with identity 3; new ethic of 18–22, 130–33; problematization of 57–9, 132; rethinking 1–2; stylization of active 115–19
'older' subjectivities 2–3
ontology of ageing 12–13

participants 46, 53; profiles **49–50**
patients, consultation with cosmetic surgeon 63
performativity, politics of 130–33
Pitts, V. 73, 89
Pitts-Taylor, V. 4, 5, 21, 80, 96
plastic surgery, cosmetic surgery *vs.* 75–6, 87
politics: as an ethics 2; of performativity 130–33; of possibility 112; of risk, ageing and 9–10; of truth 112; *see also* neoliberalism
Powell, J. L. 9–10, 107
power: Foucault and 32, 33, 129; in materiality of the body 102; self-care and 131–2; subjectivation and 5
power/knowledge 32
practices of the self 33–5, 42–3; constitution of subject through 63; cosmetic surgery and 44–5; defined 33; shaping subjective experience and 106
practitioner profiles **51–2**
premature ageing 58
problematization 53; of ageing of older body 68, 69; of anti-ageing discourse 75–9; of demographic ageing 10; of 'older' 132; of older self 57–9; of vanity 81–2; of youth in aesthetics 106–10
Probyn, E. 62, 105–6, 119
'psy' discourses, cosmetic surgery and 88–9

Rabinow, P. 30–1, 34, 36, 44, 121, 131
reflexive self-expression, ethical formation of older subject and 19
refresh 74
regimens: of power 32; of truth 32
rejuvenation 73, 74
renewal 73
're,' notion of 73, 74–5
renovation 74
reparative reading 2
reposition 74
resistance, new forms of subjectivity and ethics of 44
restoration 74
reversal 73, 74
rhinoplasty 76
risks of cosmetic surgery 66–7, 102–5
Ms Robinson (study participant): on age-appropriate cosmetic surgery 104; on ageing gracefully 101; on combination of cosmetic surgery and leisure practices 92; on cosmetic surgery and bodily maintenance 82; on cosmetic surgery and psychological health 88–9; on preventing effects of ageing 74; profile of **51**; on shift in what it means to be 'older' 121
Rose, N. 9, 10, 37, 38, 40, 86, 87

Sedgwick, E. K. 2, 105
self: authentic 21, 62–4; body as site for work on 40; enfolded relation to body 64; practices of the self 33–5, 42–3; reflexive relationship with 41; renunciation of 36
self-care: bodily maintenance and 81–8; cosmetic surgery as 19–20, 21, 73; ethic of freedom and creativity and

93–5; neoliberalism and 128; power and 131–2; virtue and 85
self-fulfillment, cosmetic surgery and 21, 81, 88–9
self-improvement 21
self-indulgence, cosmetic surgery as 21, 81, 89–92
self-stylization, cosmetic surgery as 2, 19–20, 22
self-surveillance by older people in relation to age-related norms 67–8
signification: aesthetic enhancement and 80; consumer choices and 40
Dr Smith (study participant) 75; on ageing disgracefully 110; on cosmetic surgery as autonomous choice 91; on desirable older body 109; on dissonance between chronological age and appearance 59; on growing old gracefully 101; on 'old' as state of mind 120; profile of **51**; on treatment of older persons 114
social identity, formation of 12
social movements challenging age-based discrimination 6–7, 23n3
social policies, ageing well and 19–19
social risks: of cosmetic surgery 103; posed by older people 10
social welfare: lifestyle choices and 39; young old and 118–19
socio-political regulation of ageing 9–11
Sophie (study participant): on cosmetic surgery as consumer practice 91; profile of **50**; on transgression of age-appropriate norms 110
stylization: of active 'older' self 115–19; of 'older' self 73, 112–14
subject: cosmetic surgery and becoming a 4–5; ethical principles and aesthetic relationship with 34–5; Foucault and 32–3; in games of truth 57–60; hermeneutics of 62, 63–4; relation to truth 15–16, 57–60
subjectivation 40–2, 54n2; ethical substance and 42; four folds of 20, 21; 'know yourself' and 36; mode of subjection and 42; power and 5; practice of self and 42–3; *telos* and 43–4
subjectivity: consumer 39–40; Foucault's forms of 32, 33; 'older' 2–3; resistance and new forms of 44
Sullivan, N. 105, 106
Ms Taylor (study participant): on cosmetic surgery as consumer practice 90, 91; on desirable older body 109; on dissonance between chronological age and appearance 58; on dissonance between outer expression and inner feeling 60; profile of **52**; on self-care and ageing gracefully 102; on shift in what it means to be 'older' 121; on treatment of older persons 114
techne tou biou 43
technologies of self 43
tekhne 39, 73
telos 43–4
therapeutic intervention, cosmetic surgery and 21
third age 10, 117–19
to look better, not younger 21
Tom (study participant): on age and cosmetic surgery 65; on being active 115; on bodily maintenance 83; on cosmetic surgery as autonomous choice 91; on enhancing appearance through surgery 79; on looking good for one's age 67; profile of **50**; on reasons older people have cosmetic surgery 68; on self-care 84
transformation, becoming older and 17–18
true identity 15–16
truth: authentic self and 63–4; Foucault and 32; games of 32; relation to subject 15–16
Tulle, E. 13, 106, 119
Tulle-Winton, E. 61, 107–8
Twigg, Julia 15, 31, 61, 107, 123n5

vanity, problematizing 81–2
virtue, self-care and 85

Dr Watts (study participant): on age-related change 76–7; on anti-ageing medicine 75; on cosmetic surgery as consumer practice 90; on dissonance between chronological age and appearance 59; profile of **52**; on reversing effects of ageing 74; on vanity 82
wealth, active 'older' lifestyle and 116–17
Dr Williams (study participant): on bodily maintenance 83; on normalization of cosmetic surgery 84; profile of **52**; on reversing effects of ageing 74

will to health 86
Dr Wilson (study participant): on aesthetics and cosmetic surgery 93–4; on age and cosmetic surgery 65, 66; on choice to appear 'older' 85; on chronological age and phenotypic age 119; on dissonance between chronological age and appearance 58; on dissonance between outer expression and inner feeling 60; on elderly identity 114; on enhancing appearance through surgery 79; profile of **52**; self-care and ageing gracefully 102

young old 10, 17–19
youth, problematizing in aesthetics 106–10
youthful ideals discourse 14–15

For Product Safety Concerns and Information please contact our
EU representative GPSR@taylorandfrancis.com Taylor & Francis
Verlag GmbH, Kaufingerstraße 24, 80331 München, Germany